DRAWING on the science that has made her *the* go-to expert on the connection between food and sleep, Dr. Marie-Pierre St-Onge pairs her comprehensive strategies for getting a good night's sleep with 75 recipes that work with the body's hormones and circadian rhythm to promote sleep at bedtime so you feel energetic during the day and ready for sleep at night. Satisfying and easy to prepare, these recipes follow a delicious Mediterranean diet. Here, too, is a 28-day meal plan that takes the guesswork out of what to eat when so you can start sleeping better than ever.

Eat Better, Sleep Better is for anyone who wants food to be the medicine for getting quality sleep.

The recipes include the following:

- **EASY BREAKFASTS:** Make-Ahead Morning Muffins; Overnight Oats with Ginger, Winter Compote, and Walnuts

- **SALADS AND SOUPS:** Chilled-Out Soba Salad with Edamame and Sesame-Ginger Vinaigrette; Creamy Lemon-Turkey Soup with Barley and Mint

- **SIDE DISHES AND MEATLESS MAINS:** Soy-Braised Butternut Squash with Miso Butter and Black Sesame; Mushroom "Carbonara" with Broccoli Rabe and Parmesan; Focaccia with Beefsteak Tomatoes and Olives

- **LOW-STRESS EVENING MEALS:** Portuguese-Style Tomato Rice with Mussels and Scallops; Grilled Chicken Cutlets with Midsummer Mostarda; Pan-Seared Halibut with Barley-Artichoke Risotto

- **SWEETS FOR SLEEP:** Sesame Shortbread Cookies; Easy Stone Fruit Sorbet; Chamomile-Ginger Panna Cotta with Midsummer Compote and Pistachios

Eat Better,
Sleep Better

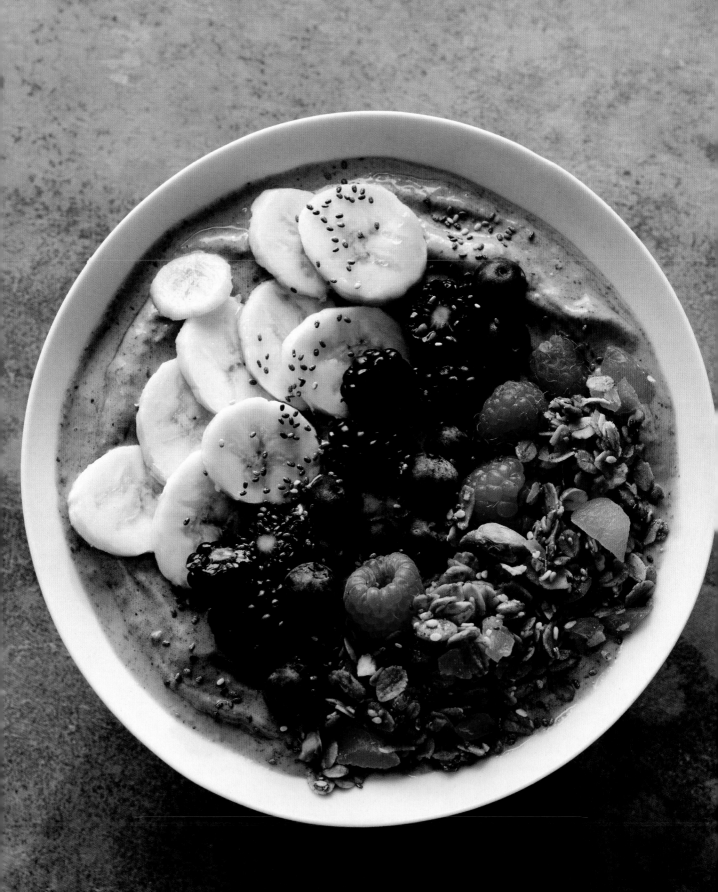

Banana-Berry Smoothie Bowl
with Chia and Granola, page 136

Eat Better, Sleep Better

75 RECIPES AND A 28-DAY MEAL PLAN
THAT UNLOCK THE FOOD-SLEEP CONNECTION

Dr. Marie-Pierre St-Onge,
PhD, CCSH, FAHA

AND

Kat Craddock

PHOTOGRAPHY BY DAVID MALOSH

SIMON ELEMENT

NEW YORK   LONDON   TORONTO   SYDNEY   NEW DELHI

SIMON
ELEMENT

An Imprint of Simon & Schuster, LLC
1230 Avenue of the Americas
New York, NY 10020

First Simon Element hardcover edition January 2025

SIMON ELEMENT is a trademark of Simon & Schuster, LLC

For information about special discounts for bulk purchases, please
contact Simon & Schuster Special Sales at 1-866-506-1949 or
business@simonandschuster.com.

The Simon & Schuster Speakers Bureau can bring authors to your
live event. For more information or to book an event, contact the
Simon & Schuster Speakers Bureau at 1-866-248-3049 or visit
our website at www.simonspeakers.com.

Interior design by Jan Derevjanik and Toni Tajima

Manufactured in China

10 9 8 7 6 5 4 3 2 1

Library of Congress Cataloging-in-Publication Data
has been applied for.

ISBN 978-1-9821-9844-2
ISBN 978-1-9821-9851-0 (ebook)

Opposite: Blackberry-Plum Galette
with a Corn Crust, page 253

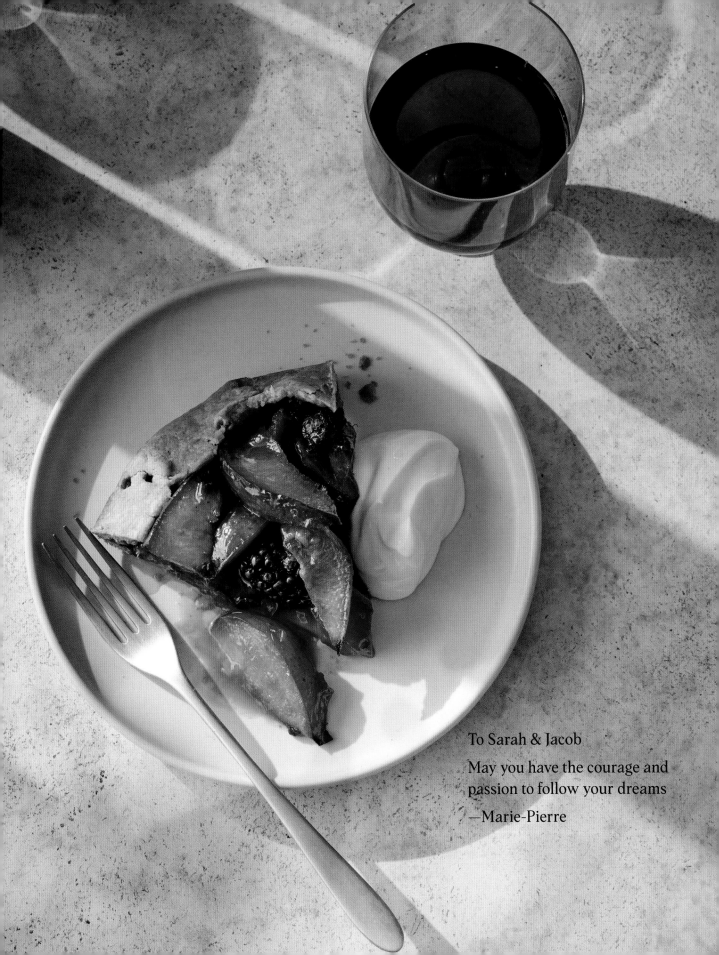

To Sarah & Jacob

May you have the courage and
passion to follow your dreams

—Marie-Pierre

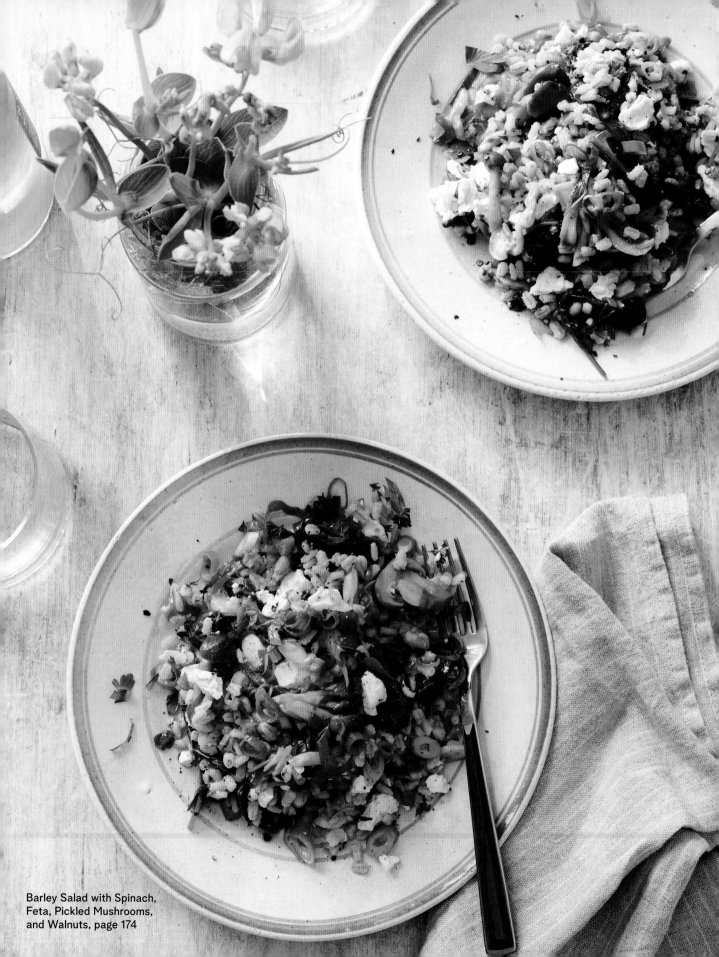

Barley Salad with Spinach,
Feta, Pickled Mushrooms,
and Walnuts, page 174

Contents

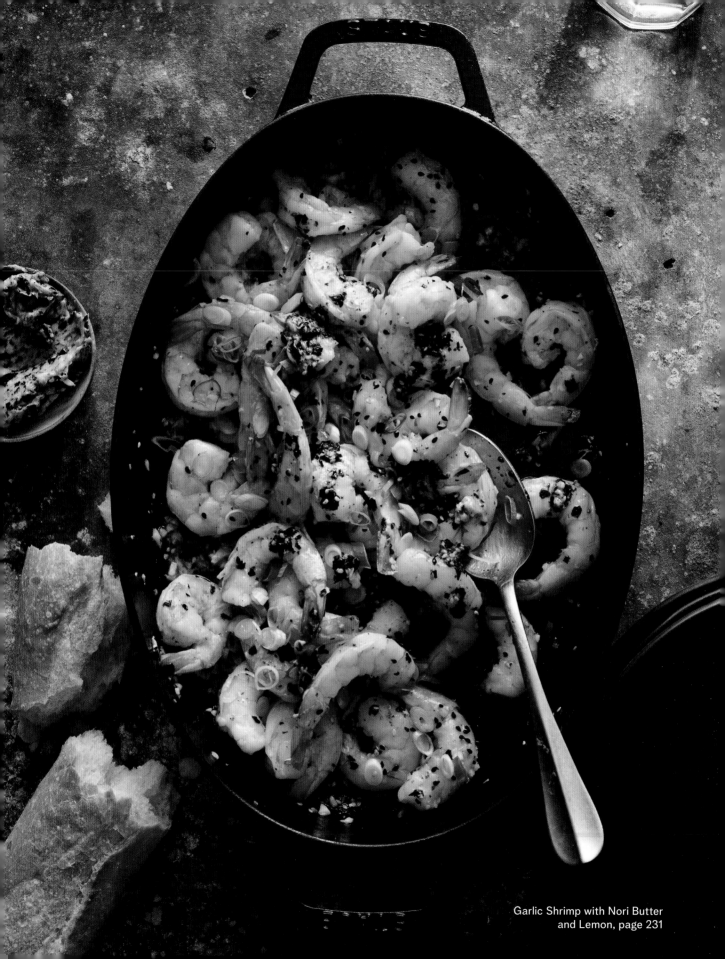

Garlic Shrimp with Nori Butter and Lemon, page 231

Foreword

Christopher Gardner, PhD,
Professor of Medicine, Stanford University

Everyone eats and everyone sleeps, every day, over their entire lifespan (with the exception of a few days here and there—perhaps an all-nighter studying for a big exam, a religious fast, a chaotic flare-up in one's schedule where food and sleep are in short supply). There is unequivocal evidence that the quality of what we eat and the quality of our sleep have a strong influence on our health and vitality. How empowering that we can make personal choices regarding eating and sleeping!

Unfortunately, many of us do not eat and/or sleep optimally. Perhaps that's why you've picked up this book. Of course, some people have more influence over their choices than others. Let's acknowledge that there are societal, environmental, geographic, political, and other factors beyond our control that may prevent us from taking full advantage of the healthier choices we would prefer to make.

But maybe one of the reasons we aren't making the best choices we can is that the many options for eating and sleeping can be confusing. When I first met Dr. Marie-Pierre St-Onge twenty years ago, we spoke at length about the strong connection she had observed between eating and sleeping. This was one of my personal aha moments. They are aligned!

Fortunately for you, dear reader, Dr. St-Onge has dedicated her career to studying this alignment. Not only does she understand the relationship from a scientific perspective, but also many of the careful studies she has conducted and published over the last twenty years have tested and defined those connections. That's precisely why she is one of the most well-known international leaders in the study of diet and sleep.

Her lifetime of research is so compelling and so important that it is no longer enough to share her findings and insights among her colleagues at scientific conferences or in academic journals. It's time to make these powerful insights accessible to a wider audience, and the result is the excellent book now in your hands.

Before you immerse yourself in these helpful pages, I'd like to share some of what I've come to know and love about Marie-Pierre. Most of my interactions with her have involved activities with the American Heart

Association (AHA). We have attended AHA's scientific meetings and held positions in its committees and councils for almost two decades. In general, the hundreds and sometimes thousands of scientists, physicians, and researchers who go to those conferences are smart and scholarly individuals who have chosen a life of research. Marie-Pierre can go toe-to-toe on scholarship on any day with any one of them, but she also has the gift of being an excellent teacher and communicator. Not every scientist has that strength.

Additionally, Marie-Pierre has a superpower rare among scholars in the world of health—she is fun and likes to have fun. This helps her to better connect with her audiences and appreciate that optimal diets and sleep patterns also must allow for optimizing joy and pleasure in life. I'm sure you are not only going to appreciate the wisdom she is sharing with you in her book but also how she delivers it.

I am a nutrition scientist and professor of medicine at Stanford University. I have served on the Nutrition Committee of the Lifestyle Council of the AHA, among others, where I spent time with Marie-Pierre. In 2016 she was the writing-chair of a critically important AHA Scientific Statement on Sleep Duration and Quality. After several years of the AHA's promoting "Life's Simple Seven"—diet, physical activity, blood pressure, blood cholesterol, blood glucose, body weight, tobacco control—sleep was added to the list in 2022. The messaging changed to "Life's Essential Eight." It came as no surprise to anyone that Marie-Pierre was instrumental to that change and will chair the newly formed Sleep Committee, in 2025. Her engagement, leadership, and productivity have been exemplary.

One of my fondest memories of working with Marie-Pierre came from our role on the planning committee for the spring 2016 AHA conference for the Epidemiology and Lifestyle Councils held in Phoenix, Arizona.

We put together a session to address the *culinary* aspect of heart-healthy food, and the roles that home cooks and chefs could play in our efforts to help Americans eat more healthfully. The guest speakers included a chef, a food ethnographer, and the vice president of Strategic Initiatives and Industry Leadership at the Culinary Institute of America. Together they discussed the importance of including taste in communications and approaches that promoted a heart-healthy diet. They referred to this in terms of "craveability" and "unapologetic deliciousness."

The reaction of the thousand-plus scientists attending the session was overwhelmingly positive. This was a topic, and a style of presentation, that was very different than the usual charts, graphs, hypotheses, and conclusions that attendees were accustomed to viewing at the conference. This collaboration with Marie-Pierre was immensely gratifying for me, particularly because I was teaming up with a card-carrying PhD scientist who shared my interest in seeking nontraditional approaches to promoting health messaging.

Marie-Pierre has served on many national committees and received dozens of awards for her scholarship, including some of science's most prestigious, such as the Fulbright. No dry academic, Marie-Pierre is fun-loving and hard-working, a mother and wife, and someone who really practices what she preaches. She maintains a stable sleep schedule and gets at least seven hours of sleep each night. She eats a plant-forward diet and loves to cook. She is an avid cyclist who rides her bike to work every day and coaches her kids' mountain bike team. She has completed fourteen marathons, including the Boston Marathon—three times! Marie-Pierre is an inspiration to all who come to know and love her.

It was never part of her long-term plan to write a book for a lay audience, but she has always been passionate about sharing her deep knowledge and understanding of nutrition and sleep with others. She is a true pioneer in this space. Although the connections between what we eat and how we sleep may seem obvious, very few scientists study this directly. Fortunately, Marie-Pierre has made this her life's work.

Her findings and her communication of this field of science will empower you intellectually and practically to make positive changes in your health and for your life. After digesting this book and perhaps sleeping on it, puns intended, you will eat better, sleep better, and enjoy a healthier, happier, and more vibrant you.

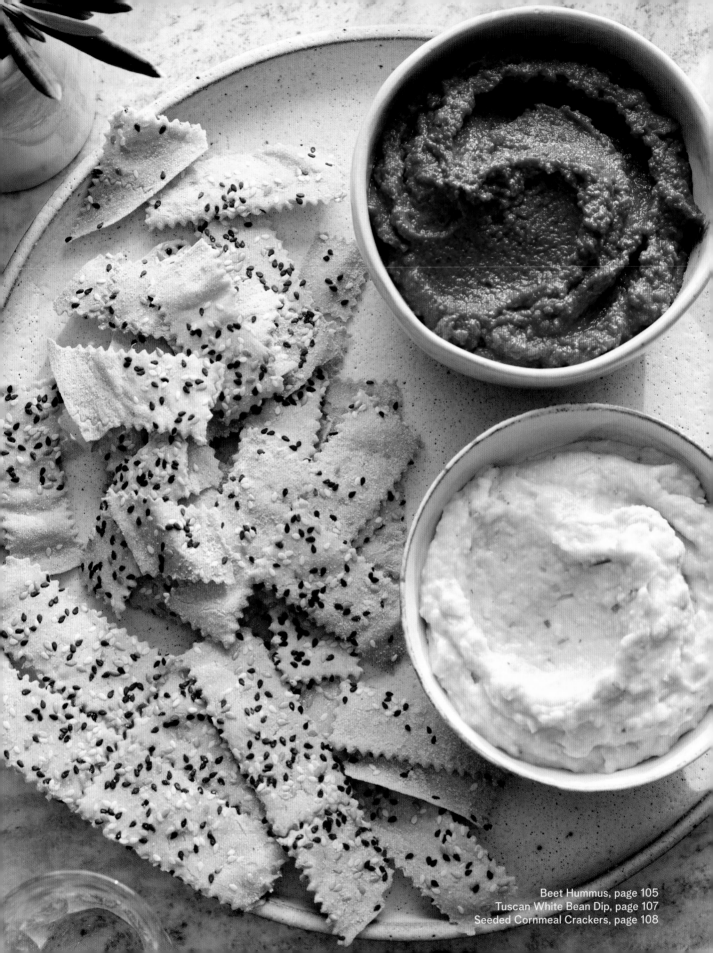

Beet Hummus, page 105
Tuscan White Bean Dip, page 107
Seeded Cornmeal Crackers, page 108

Introduction

If you eat better, you will sleep better—it's as simple as that. And if you sleep better, you'll be healthier, and you'll enjoy many more days (and nights) on this planet.

Without good sleep, our bodies—especially our brains—stay tired and can't recuperate. As a result, we get sick much more easily. Our immune system is weakened, which increases the risk for a host of acute and chronic illnesses that can affect nearly every organ system, from our brain and heart to our gut and skin and everything in between.

Lousy sleep increases our vulnerability to disorders such as hypertension, gastrointestinal problems, and even catching a common cold—and it makes us more prone to weight gain and other cardiometabolic disorders like type 2 diabetes and cardiovascular disease. In other words, poor sleep and poor diet are the drivers of a vicious cycle in our brains and bodies: When we're tired, we frequently reach for foods that are higher in sugar and saturated fat (and calories). The result is unwanted weight gain, which can lead to a range of health issues, from sleep apnea to serious cardiovascular problems.

Sleep issues also contribute to stress and anxiety, as well as poor decision-making. Have you ever tried to write an important email or text, or read and process crucial information when you're exhausted?

> When we're tired, we frequently reach for foods that are higher in sugar and saturated fat (and calories).

Participate in an important discussion at work or at home or make financial (or any other important) decisions? It's much easier to make thoughtful choices when you're well-rested. When you're sleep-deprived, your decision-making abilities can be compromised even when you're doing something on autopilot, such as driving home from work. If you're not alert, you might miss even a familiar stop sign and drive right through it.

Mental health problems and cognitive disorders, such as depression and Alzheimer's disease, have also been linked to a lack of good-quality sleep. And while Alzheimer's disease typically develops in older age, mental health can be compromised by poor sleep at any age. The American Academy of Pediatrics reports that sleep disorders in adolescents are associated with problems ranging from depression to poor cognitive performance in school.

Bottom line? It's not just our physical well-being that hinges on having good sleep quality. Our mental well-being is affected as well.

Unfortunately, we are battling an epidemic of sleep deprivation. In the U.S. alone, about 70 million people report some form of sleep disorder, and while there are many reasons for our restless nights, my research has led me to conclude that our diets—what we eat, and what we don't—play a major role.

As a nutrition scientist and researcher at Columbia University, I've conducted extensive research on the relationship among food, sleep, and health, and I keep coming back to one conclusion: If you make some easy (and great-tasting) fixes to your diet, you will sleep better. And when you improve the quality of sleep you get, you'll lower your risk factors for disease and improve your overall health.

This sleep-diet connection is life-changing—perhaps even life-saving—news, and I'm about to give you an original, simple method for incorporating it into your days and, most importantly, improving the quality of your nights.

Why I Want to Help You Eat and Sleep Better

I'm keenly aware of the connection between our health and our quality of life. Without one, it's difficult to maintain the other—and if you've had even the slightest brush with any illness, you know this equilibrium is key. I grew up seeing the devastating impact of heart disease on my father's family, particularly among his siblings who suffered from high cholesterol and blood pressure. Unfortunately, my dad did as well. In fact, as a teenager I wanted to become a heart surgeon. While I did not go this route, my research revolves around heart disease.

Despite his healthy lifestyle, my dad couldn't escape his genetic predisposition for heart disease. As a preventive measure, on his doctor's advice, my dad started taking cholesterol-reducing statins in his 40s. He also wanted to do something to help others at high risk for cardio-vascular disease, or CVD, and he became a faithful fundraiser for the Heart and Stroke Foundation of Canada, where I grew up. Because of my father, I was aware of the dangers of CVD—which still kills more Americans every year than all forms of cancer combined. And because of the example he set, I wanted to do something to help, as well.

When I was studying nutrition at McGill University, my father asked me if there were foods he could eat that would help him become less reliant on his medications. He was ahead of his time seeing food as the best medicine for reducing and controlling his cholesterol through eating well rather than simply popping a pill. He knew about the connection between diet and heart health, of course, but wanted a deeper level of information—action steps he could take. A handful of cherries with breakfast? Some walnuts or almonds for an afternoon snack?

"I'd rather drink kefir, than take a daily pill," he'd say casually in anticipation of my findings. I was researching fermented dairy products, which have anti-inflammatory properties that can lower the risk of heart disease. It wasn't quite as simple as drinking kefir, and I would never have advised him to stop his statins. Still, my father was on the right track, drawing a straight line from what he ate to how he felt, and his questions were always in the back of my mind.

When people hear that I'm a professor of nutritional medicine, many ask some variation of my dad's questions. "What can I eat to control my blood pressure?" "What foods are good for quick energy?" "Can I lower my risk of cancer by eating certain foods?" "What nutrients will boost my immune system during flu season?" "Can I protect my cognitive function through diet?" "What should I eat to lose weight?" I often also get "What do *you* eat?"

Whatever questions you can come up with about "prescribing" food for health issues, I've probably heard them. And as a scientist, I've addressed variations of them through my research on *functional foods*—those foods that go beyond meeting our nutritional needs and offer quantifiable health benefits, like lowering the risk of disease and even improving our quality of life as we age.

> Functional foods are those foods that go beyond meeting our nutritional needs and offer quantifiable health benefits.

Here are just a handful of examples of what functional foods are, and what they have to offer. Legumes—from chickpeas to lentils to red beans—are high in fiber and are a great source of muscle-building lean protein; olive oil provides healthy fat with anti-inflammatory properties that benefit every body system; tart cherries contain complex carbohydrates that pack a lot of fiber into a small, tasty package; walnuts and almonds deliver essential nutrients like zinc and magnesium, as well as protein, fiber, and healthy fat. Beyond their nutritional content, these foods are part of health claims to reduce the risk of various diseases, including CVD. There are many more examples you'll find on our plan on page 85, including anti-inflammatory fermented foods like that tangy kefir my father was so keen to try.

So what does nutrition have to do with getting a good night's sleep? We know that while poor nutrition is indeed a primary risk factor for heart disease, depression and anxiety, diabetes, and other life-threatening medical conditions, *poor sleep also plays a major role in determining how and why we get sick.* There is a proven link between the nutritional value of the food we eat, the quality of the sleep we get, and our health. If we eat well, we sleep well, and we can enjoy good health. The opposite is also true.

I've shown how skimping on sleep leads people to eat more than they may need, and why a lack of sleep can stimulate the networks in our brains that are involved in the "food reward" mindset. When we're tired, we tend to choose foods not based on what our bodies need (or even if we're genuinely hungry), but on what we want in the moment—a quick hit of pleasure, a food we "deserve," perhaps because we're exhausted. Think of it this way: A tired brain and body will steer you to a "reward" of a fast-food fried apple pie, not an apple. People in one of my studies ate about 300 more calories and consumed 33 percent more saturated fat when they slept too little compared to when they slept well. That was after four nights of limited sleep. Imagine what happens to our overall health when we do that for weeks, months, and years on end. (Interestingly, Esra Tasali, MD, director of the Sleep Research Center at the University of Chicago, and her colleagues have shown that increasing sleep leads people to eat about 270 *fewer* calories per day.)

I'll explain my work more thoroughly throughout this book, but for now, consider this fact: Though it starts differently for every person, the vicious cycle of bad sleep and bad diet can go round and round, with devastating consequences.

I am going to give you a simple way to stop it, for good.

Functional Foods: The Way to Break the Sick-and-Tired Cycle

Eat Better, Sleep Better isn't about sipping chamomile tea before going to bed in your cool, dark bedroom as you fall asleep to the sounds of a white-noise app. Although good sleep practices—a consistent sleep-wake schedule, a comfortable environment, a wind-down routine before bed, and other proven sleep-enhancing behaviors and elements—are key to a good night's sleep, at the heart of my plan you'll find delicious meals that lean into functional foods you'll consume throughout the day (note that point about "throughout the day"—it will come up again) so you can

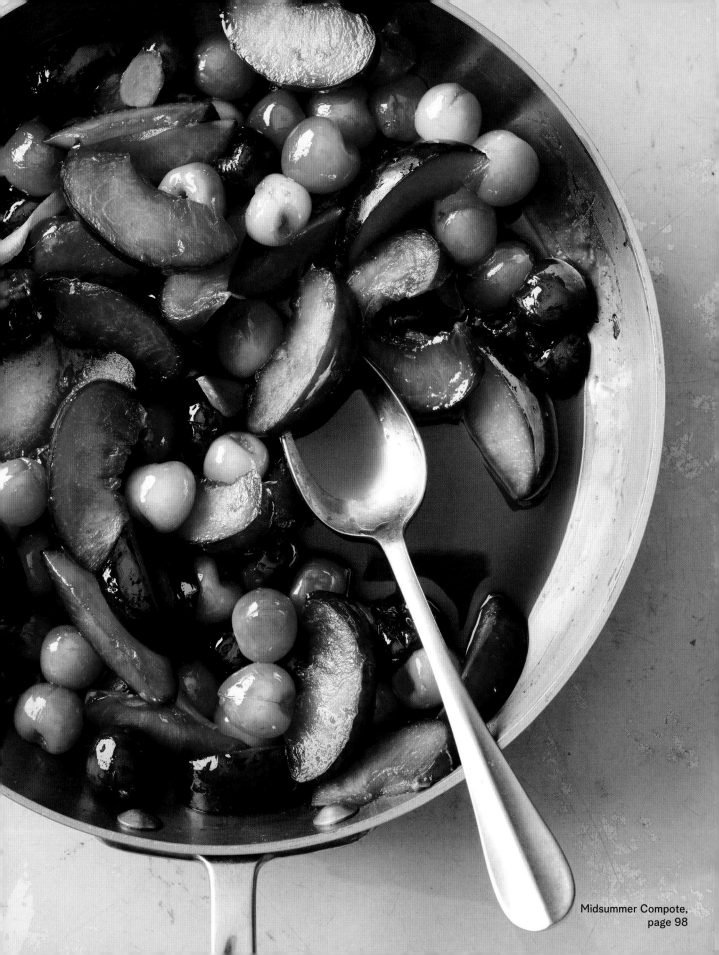

Midsummer Compote,
page 98

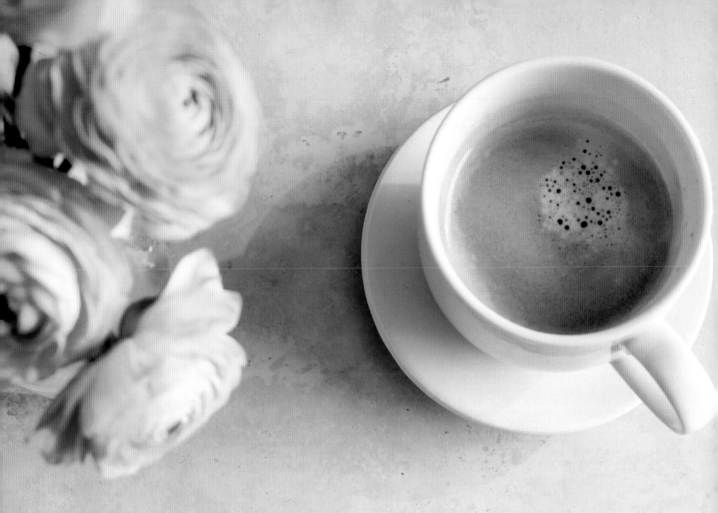

A Note on the Research

Throughout *Eat Better, Sleep Better*, I'll refer to clinical intervention studies, many of which are the result of years of work by my team of research assistants, fellows, graduate students, and colleagues. Sleep-focused nutrition science is explored by a small but mighty community of scientists (both PhDs and MDs) supported by well-trained research assistants, laboratory technicians, and trainees. New findings are published regularly. I'll also cite a number of studies conducted by my colleagues in the field that have been either foundational to or supportive of my own research.

My work mostly involves two different styles of research conducted in humans: clinical intervention studies and population studies.

Clinical intervention studies (my specific area of expertise) enroll a small number of participants, usually between 10 and 30 people, and assign participants to an intervention, like a specific diet, to test various health effects. Actual sample sizes for these studies depend on the specific outcome (or health measure) being tested and the level of control included in the intervention. For example, a smaller number is needed for inpatient studies, when individuals are studied in a clinical environment under well-controlled conditions, than for outpatient studies, when people participate from home and live their lives more freely.

I also use data from population studies to test associations between various lifestyle factors, like diet and sleep quality, and health. These studies usually include hundreds to thousands of participants representing various gender, age, and racial groups. It's important to note that regardless of the type of study we conduct, we are always assessing group effects, not individual effects, to allow us to extrapolate findings to guide recommendations for a larger population. So, while I can't necessarily pinpoint a food or ingredient that was particularly helpful for one person or another, I can evaluate patterns that were helpful for the group in general.

get the best sleep of your life at night. And *the secret is how and when to combine these foods strategically*, to optimize the messages your brain sends to your body. I'll explain this more in the chapters to come, but here is what you need to know now:

As soon as you swallow a bite of food and it enters your system, your brain goes to work, running its own intel on the components of that food. Let's assume what you're eating has one or some of the following sleep-supporting nutrients: the amino acid tryptophan, magnesium, zinc, and certain B vitamins. These are essential catalysts for sleep, but they won't work on their own. (And you can't trick your brain with supplements.) However, if throughout the day you *combine* foods containing these nutrients (specifically protein-rich foods with healthy, fiber-rich carbohydrates), the ensuing chemical reactions will help you fall asleep faster and stay asleep. The food in *Eat Better, Sleep Better* will trigger the brain to synthesize two must-have, sleep-supporting hormones: melatonin and serotonin.

To sum it up? Choose the right foods during the day, and you'll get a great night's sleep.

How to Use This Book

If you want to skip straight to the food lists and recipes in *Eat Better, Sleep Better*, you can do so, but I suggest you read through the chapters that precede them. You'll be more invested in my approach to eating if you understand the why-it-works before you dive into the how-to-do-it. That is why the first few chapters cover topics like the science of the sleep-food connection, including my ongoing research on its link to the overall health of your heart, and your arteries—all of which affect your brain health and the health and working order of virtually every other system in your body. Doctors call this cardiometabolic health, and it is the cornerstone of overall health and well-being.

I'll demystify the sleep hormones melatonin and serotonin, both of which we naturally produce but that can be boosted by different foods, especially those containing tryptophan, the essential amino acid that can turn foods like turkey into a sleep aid. (Of course, there's more to it than that, but the link among tryptophan, serotonin, and melatonin is one you'll be reading lots about.)

You'll learn about the four must-have nutrients for sleep, and you'll get a master list of sleep-supporting foods, along with a 28-day plan for resetting your sleep cycle. Along the way, you'll discover tips for improving your sleep quality at every age and stage of your life; how to troubleshoot sleep disorders like insomnia, as well as sleep disruptors such as traveling across time zones (which results in jet lag); and why maintaining healthy circadian rhythms—your body's optimal times for various processes, including digestion and alertness—is essential. (You'll also find a resource section at the back of the book on some sleep and food topics.) When you're ready, it's time to get cooking (and eating!) for better sleep.

Worried that I'm going to ask you to eat weird things that are hard to prepare, taste like cardboard, or are expensive to shop for? Or that I'm going to tell you to eliminate all caffeine effective immediately and go on a juice cleanse? Not at all! This isn't about deprivation or a hard-to-follow program. I live in the real world like you (and like to indulge in a treat once in a while), juggling work and family . . . all the more reason to want good-quality sleep!

You may be feeding yourself or a whole crew. Perhaps you need portable snacks or a grab-and-go breakfast, foods you can pack for lunch at work, or dinners that your family will enjoy, too. Maybe you need make-ahead items and would like to have freezable leftovers, both of which would make life easier. (Aren't leftovers the best?)

I've anticipated all that, which is why my eating plan is very much about adding great, easy-to-make meals and snacks to your lineup, and wonderful sleep-supporting staples to your pantry, rather than taking things away or turning your kitchen upside down. True, there are some foods, including processed fatty foods and products with refined sugar, that impede the quest for quality sleep (and I'll explain why that is). And as you already know, those foods don't contribute to your health in other ways, either. I'll help you find ways to avoid those foods by steering you toward healthier alternatives. And my hunch is that achieving better sleep at night will help make it even easier to make better dietary choices!

You'll find more than 75 fantastic recipes created by my co-author Kat Craddock, a former chef and renowned recipe developer and food writer. Kat has put her extensive knowledge and appreciation of good food into our easy-to-follow 28-day plan that will help you get the sleep you need. Her recipes are so delicious and accessible that you'll likely go well beyond 28 days and incorporate them into your repertoire. Best of all are the additional benefits to following an eat-better, sleep-better plan. You'll naturally lower your inflammation levels, decrease your stress, improve your cardiovascular health, and, if it's a goal of yours, you may also shed a few pounds.

Kat's easy-to-prepare yet absolutely delicious recipes cleverly incorporate sleep-supporting ingredients into everyday meals. For example, start your morning with our easy-to-make ginger-infused take on overnight oats (page 132) or Make-Ahead Morning Muffins (bake and freeze a batch) (page 150). For lunch, enjoy a Chilled Out Soba Salad with Edamame and Sesame-Ginger Vinaigrette (page 165) or a savory barley salad (page 174). Dinner can be Lemony Baked Trout (page 220) or Chickpea Gemelli with Butternut Squash, Walnuts, and Parmesan (page 194). Make ahead and mix and match to suit your own needs and tastes.

Preparing and enjoying nourishing, delicious food and sharing it with friends and family is incredibly satisfying. So is getting a good night's sleep and waking up feeling restored and energized all day long, which, in turn, will provide you with the energy and motivation to prepare healthy and sleep-supporting meals regularly. Eating and sleeping are both essential for our well-being and our survival. But why not think of these basic human necessities as pleasures we deserve? You'll be more motivated to take care of yourself and your loved ones as you take steps to nourish and rest your body and brain.

I'm well aware that I can't eliminate all the things that have you tossing and turning, but I know that I can help you get on an excellent, science-based path to reclaiming the healing sleep you need each night, beginning with what you eat during the day.

Let's get started! My wish for you: Eat, sleep, and be healthy.

—Marie-Pierre St-Onge, PhD,
Columbia University

Part 1

Good Food, Good Sleep, Good Health

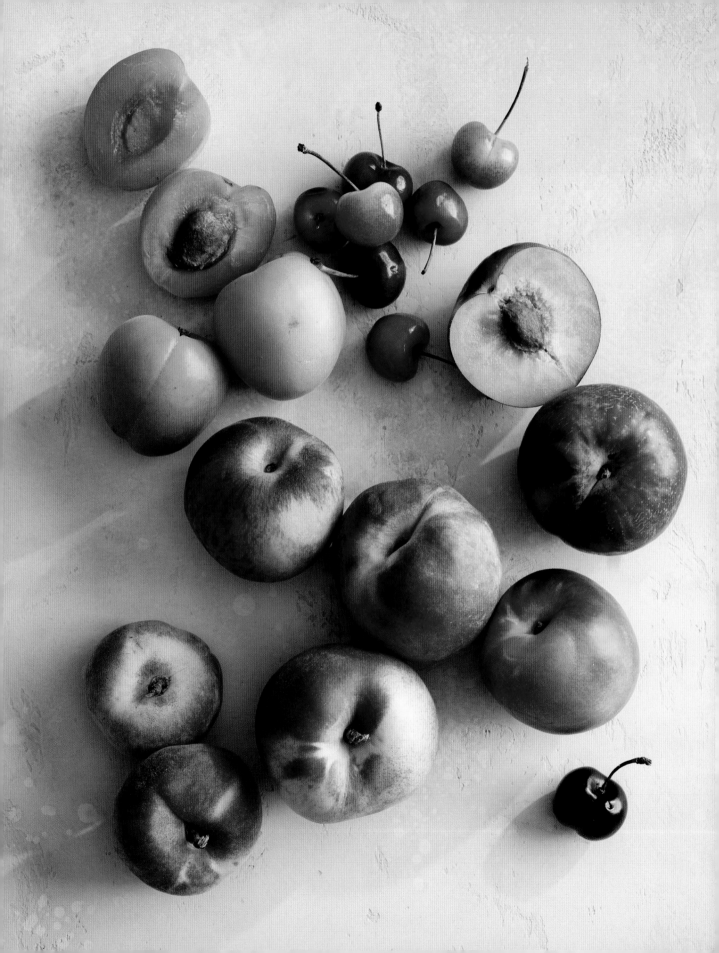

Chapter 1

How Food Can Solve Your Sleep Problems

Who hasn't experienced bad sleep at some point in their life? Maybe you were tossing and turning over a job or a relationship. Maybe a new baby was keeping you up or you were worrying about your aging parents. Perhaps your partner was snoring or kicking you awake because *you* were snoring! Or you woke up to use the bathroom three hours after you fell asleep because you drank a giant glass of water too close to bedtime. Then you got back into bed and your mind started racing about your work, relationship, baby, parents, or your restless partner. And then you started stressing about not getting enough sleep. We've all been there.

While there are innumerable everyday problems and stressors that can keep you up at night, it is also true that, like any health concern, diet plays an essential role in reversing, or at least ameliorating, illness, and what you eat is an essential part of improving your sleep health. There are specific foods that will help you fall asleep at night—and stay asleep. And, conversely, poor food choices, likely resulting from the bad sleep you've had, contribute to sleeplessness.

There's a direct link between what we eat and how we sleep, and I've been researching it for years.

When "sleep health" started to gain momentum as an important aspect of 21st century self-care, some sleep scientists and doctors called out the sleep-food connection, though I'd been encountering it in my findings for years. The commonsense recommendations they offered to desperately tired folks were good but not really groundbreaking: no caffeine after 4:00 P.M., no heavy meals or rich food too close to bedtime, and limit alcohol at night. In addition, the chronically sleep deprived were advised to "unplug" from all screens at least an hour before going to bed, to avoid too many liquids close to bedtime, to use blackout shades and white-noise machines, and to keep the bedroom cool.

There's a direct link between what we eat and how we sleep

This is certainly helpful advice, but may not be enough to solve a growing epidemic of bad sleep, and the resulting bad health outcomes. As I considered my own findings, I had to wonder: *Why aren't we looking into the sleep-food/food-sleep connection from a diet point of view?* I figured it was likely because most people, from the sleep-deprived to the researchers, were focused on fixing a sleep problem, not looking for a food solution. And why would they? Much of the research on sleep was conducted by sleep medicine experts, not nutrition scientists like me. But the connections (and solution) are clear.

Imagine a triangle with "health" at the top. On the base, you have "food" as one point and "sleep" as the other.

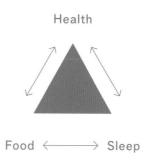

The well-established health-food link was a given in science, and the sleep-health link was backed by research as well. But the sleep-food link, evident to me and the few other nutrition and sleep scientists researching this question, was equally important. Based on the science, there is no doubt: Quality sleep and optimal health are enhanced by a nutritious, balanced diet. The reverse is also true: Poor-quality sleep and health issues are triggered or made worse by a poor diet.

Eventually, another key finding emerged from my research: *Getting good sleep is vital for cardiometabolic health.* Cardiometabolic health—meaning the health of your heart, arteries, and body—is the foundation of overall good health, including brain function. It's now possible to connect all three points of the triangle: good food, good sleep, good health.

And it's time to turn our research into a real-world solution for anyone in search of better sleep and health, achievable through a better, sleep-supporting diet.

Making the Food-Sleep-Health Connection

It happens to everyone.

Just a few nights of tossing and turning will cause you to feel tired from the moment you drag yourself out of bed. Breakfast is coffee and toast or a bowl of sugary cereal and some juice—it's quick and you're already running late. Lunch is at your desk: a bland sandwich, some salty chips, a bottle of sweetened iced tea. More coffee. You drag in the late afternoon and crave something sweet to give you energy until you can get home. The source is often vending-machine cookies or your emergency candy bar. You're so tired when you walk through the front door, but you have to eat dinner. Pizza delivery. Stuffed crust, but a side salad, or diet soda, to make it "healthy." A few hours later, you slide into bed. And stare at the ceiling.

When the alarm goes off, it feels as if you just fell asleep, and you wake up tired once more. And even if you do manage to eat a little better today or get in a workout, you are caught up in a cycle of bad sleep and poor food choices, likely reaching for sugary, processed foods that boost energy before causing you to crash.

On top of this cycle, stress creeps in and starts to take hold. You're tired and therefore aren't as efficient or productive as you would like to be. But you're also stressed out and you feel like you should go on overdrive and "power through" your day. Yet, you still seem to be falling behind or not performing as well as you want to, at work and at home. The longer this goes on, the more areas of your life are impacted. Everything from your job performance to your personal relationships and, of course, your health takes a hit—especially your cardiometabolic health. Exhaustion and stress are a one-two punch and left unaddressed can put you at risk for heart disease, including heart attack and stroke.

When our study participants had a diet of mostly fiber and healthy fats, they enjoyed better sleep.

All too often, the trigger for poor food choices is . . . you guessed it, poor sleep, creating a downward health spiral. Health issues ranging from diabetes, stroke, and vascular dementia can be traced to poor cardiometabolic health, as can a host of conditions caused by inflammation, such as arthritis and inflammatory bowel disease.

Sometimes we are tempted to think that as we age, chronic disease will inevitably find us. But so many health problems are entirely preventable, and diet is often the key factor. And if you have genetic predispositions, how you live your life, including what (and when) you eat, how much you exercise, and how well you sleep, can help mitigate the risk.

As a nutrition scientist, I see how everyday food choices can set us up for a lifetime of good (or bad) health, and I've observed the major impact that sleep has on our food choices. As a researcher I have proof that the brain behaves very differently when you are tired.

Your brain needs good sleep . . . and good food

We know this because when my team and I used functional magnetic resonance imaging (fMRI) to study the brain under different amounts of sleep, we saw how the regions of the brain, those areas associated with processing hunger signals, behaved differently in people when they were well rested compared to when they were sleep-deprived.

When study participants were well rested—four nights of about 7.5 hours of sleep—the regions of the brain involved in cognitive control (processing information to make thoughtful choices) were activated when we showed pictures of unhealthy foods such as doughnuts, candy bars, and pizza.

But, when participants were sleep-restricted—four nights of less than four hours of sleep—the activity in response to these same pictures shifted dramatically to the brain's "reward center," the regions associated with the processing of hunger, desire, and reward.

When the human brain is sleep-deprived, it essentially triggers a hunger response and tells the body to satisfy itself with a reward—perhaps it's the appeal of a treat or comfort food. This happens even when the body doesn't need energy (calories) to survive.

Unfortunately, the reward itself tends to be high in calories—and usually loaded with sugar and saturated fat—and low in nutritional value, and chances are it will disrupt sleep. In this same study of 26 participants (half were female, half were male), we provided healthy meals, but also offered participants grocery-shopping money for them to purchase their own foods, with some individuals choosing foods high in sugar, sodium, and saturated fat.

Those who ate more sugar and refined carbohydrates (like your white bread and white pasta) had increased transitions from deeper to lighter sleep during the night (deep sleep is essential; see page 29). Additionally, those who ate more saturated fat, such as some of those "reward" foods the sleepy brain craves, had less deep sleep. When you get less deep sleep and suffer from daytime drowsiness, you are more likely to make poor food choices in a quest for quick pick-me-ups or comfort foods, and then you are back to the beginning of the vicious cycle.

Consider how this translates in everyday life, when you're standing in front of the refrigerator or pushing a cart through your local grocery store, and you haven't slept well in weeks. Frozen dinner that you can microwave? Or fresh salmon that needs to be cooked? Oatmeal that needs to be prepared and fresh fruit that needs to be cleaned and cut?

Or a box of processed, artificially flavored breakfast cereal or instant cereal? Chocolate chip cookies or a handful of almonds? Note: I'm not giving you a "good foods/bad foods" list here—just making the point that when you're tired, you're likely to reach for the quick fix. That's only human. But it's also unhealthy and can easily become a habit.

Fortunately, when our study participants had a diet with more fiber and healthy fats rather than one that was heavy with sugar and saturated fat, they enjoyed better sleep at night—less restless and deeper, more restful sleep. And when participants were well rested and we showed them pictures of unhealthy foods, the brain regions that lit up were those involved in cognitive control, suggesting they could resist those "reward" foods more easily.

The concluding evidence is stark: When people are tired, their brain leads them to unhealthy foods; when they are rested, the part of the brain that would normally drive unhealthy cravings is less active, which would lead people to reach for nutritious food, rather than what is essentially junk food—or food with "empty" calories.

Bottom line? Eating a healthful diet can set you up for better sleep at night, and having better sleep at night makes it easier for you to make healthy food choices.

In the pages that follow, we'll provide you with an eating plan that will satisfy your body (and your taste buds) and rest your brain so that you can get some shut-eye. But first, let's look more closely at a few other factors that impact both the quality and the quantity of sleep you get.

The Importance of Deep Sleep

Normal, healthy sleep does not unfold as a single, uniform process. Instead, we go through, ideally, four to five sleep cycles per night, each lasting about 90 minutes. These cycles range from light sleep to deep sleep to REM (rapid eye movement) sleep and back again. And cycles early in the night differ from those later in the night. The early cycles contain more deep sleep and less REM sleep, while those later at night contain more REM and less deep sleep. That's the normal nightly variation in sleep.

REM sleep is when we dream—it's when our brains are most active. On a sleep report (generated by a sleep study in a lab) our brains look "awake." But fear not, we're paralyzed during this sleep stage, a state that ensures we don't act out our dreams.

Deep sleep (also categorized as slow-wave sleep) is essential for health because it's when all our systems, including our immune system, can rest and repair on a molecular and cellular level. Unlike REM sleep, it's very hard to wake someone up from a deep sleep stage, and if we do wake from deep sleep, we tend to be groggier than if we're coming out of light or REM sleep. When we talk about the "healing powers of sleep," it's not just an expression—the body literally heals while we sleep, but it happens during the deepest sleep cycles. This is why staying asleep long enough to cycle through deep and REM sleep is so essential for our health.

Darkness and Light: Understanding Sleep Regulation

Here's a bit of sleep science that's worth staying awake for.

Our sleep is governed by two distinct systems: the *homeostatic system* and the *circadian system*. Our homeostatic system dictates that sleep pressure (or, simply put, sleepiness) builds up gradually over time spent awake. Think of it this way—the longer you stay awake, the sleepier you get. At the same time, our circadian system, which is regulated by exposure to light and darkness, ensures that we'll fall asleep at a time that's appropriate for us humans—and we've evolved over millennia to "choose" nighttime as the right time.

If all goes according to plan, meaning that no external factors are interfering with these processes (such as working the graveyard shift or trying to fall asleep when it's still light outside [like in summer if you live where sunsets are extremely late]), sleep pressure builds up as the day evolves, courtesy of the homeostatic system. At the same time, the circadian system helps you fight sleepiness until the time is right to lay down your head: It keeps you awake until light gradually turns to dark (i.e., after sundown). The circadian system is also what keeps you asleep through the night, even after you've slept off some of that sleep pressure. This is why night-shift workers struggle to get quality sleep during the day. They may *feel* sleep pressure, but their circadian system is telling them that the sun's still out, stay awake!

To run smoothly, both the homeostatic and circadian systems depend on a careful balance of two naturally occurring substances in the body: the hormone *melatonin* and the neurotransmitter *serotonin*. Interestingly, the essential amino acid tryptophan is at the root of these factors. That means that what we eat can optimize—or disrupt—the whole cycle. I'll explain this next.

Melatonin and serotonin

No doubt you've heard of melatonin—if only because melatonin *supplements* are a popular self-care topic and your local drugstore likely features it prominently. Supplemental melatonin, however, is not the same as the melatonin that your body regularly produces. In healthy individuals, naturally occurring melatonin levels rise in the bloodstream a few hours before bedtime, in response to darkness, signaling to the brain that it's time to give in to rising sleep pressure and go to bed.

Because this release is triggered in part by our exposure to dimming light and darkness, its secretion is hindered when we're in the presence of bright lights—including blue lights from computer, cell phone, and TV screens. (This is why sleep experts tell you to cut your screen use at least one hour before bedtime and to get those screens out of your bedroom.) Daylight saving time and flying across time zones also interfere with melatonin production. (This is where blackout shades and sleep masks come in handy, and why frequent fliers pop melatonin supplements to combat jet lag, though such supplements aren't always the answer, as you'll learn.)

You've also probably heard of serotonin, the so-called feel-good hormone. Serotonin is a neurotransmitter, meaning that it facilitates communication across the brain and body. (Neurotransmitters are a class of naturally occurring chemical compounds, made up of specific amino acids, that allow the brain to tell the body what to do, via the central nervous system that governs every aspect of human behavior. *Run faster to catch your bus. Call your mother. Hold your knife to butter your toast. Turn the page. Smile. Hit send. Remember your 4:00 P.M. meeting.*) Serotonin is a power player, exerting control on a wide range of bodily functions such as digestion and blood clotting, as well as emotional well-being, the ability to focus, sexual desire, hunger, and much more—including sleep. Low serotonin levels are associated with poor sleep, depression and mood swings, and physical ailments including gastrointestinal (GI) problems. In fact, serotonin, while produced in the brain, can also be found in the GI tract, where it transmits signals related to anxiety, hunger, and satiety to the central nervous system. This is why you may feel queasy in your belly when you're anxious.

Like melatonin, serotonin plays a major role in the various processes needed for waking and sleeping. Think of it as a controller of the duration and intensity of wakefulness, as well as a trigger for the neurological events that lead to sleep. *But our bodies can't produce adequate melatonin without producing serotonin first.* When the level of either of those is thrown off balance—for instance, by activities like staying up all night or sleeping until noon, for whatever reason—sleep is negatively impacted, and poor sleep can lead to poor health.

The good news is that there is a way to protect and optimize our internal melatonin and serotonin production with food—specifically, foods that provide tryptophan.

Tryptophan

You've likely heard someone comment about eating Thanksgiving dinner and falling asleep right after because turkey contains something mysterious called *tryptophan*—which some people think of as a kind of savory sedative. (Maybe we fall asleep after Thanksgiving dinner because we cooked all day, it's stuffy inside, the football game got boring, we overindulged and did some day drinking, and . . . someone else can clean the kitchen.) Yes, turkey has a lot of tryptophan, but so do many other foods.

Here's what tryptophan is and is not. And let's sort this out now, because many of the recipes and foods we recommend in *Eat Better, Sleep Better* are chock-full of tryptophan, for very good reasons, but also contain other important nutrients:

- **Tryptophan is an essential amino acid.** Amino acids (as you may remember from high school science) are the building blocks of all the proteins in our body that support life-sustaining biological functions. We need amino acids for tasks such as cell repair and reproduction, including blood cells and muscle tissue; for the breakdown and digestion of food, as well as gut health; for brain health, including the synthesis of neurotransmitters (such as serotonin); for heart health; for the production of enzymes and hormones (including melatonin); and more.

  There are 20 amino acids in total, but nine of them, including tryptophan, are considered essential amino acids, meaning that our bodies cannot produce them. Instead, we must get these vital compounds from food. Only foods that contain protein, including animal products such as meat, fish, and dairy, and certain plant foods can provide amino acids. When we eat these foods, the digestive enzymes in our gut go to work. They eventually break down the proteins into separate amino acids that hitch a ride in the bloodstream, traveling to different areas in the body where they are needed as building blocks for vital components such as muscle tissue, neurotransmitters, and hormones.

- **Tryptophan is necessary for the production of serotonin and melatonin.** More than 90 percent of the dietary tryptophan we consume is absorbed into the bloodstream, just like any other essential amino acid. But a fraction of what's left makes its way into the brain—*and once in the brain, dietary tryptophan is converted into serotonin and melatonin.*

- **Tryptophan is not a sedative.** It is, however, a sleep-supporting compound because it is the base from which serotonin and melatonin are produced. Eating tryptophan-rich foods *throughout the day*, not just at night, will enable a healthy sleep cycle. Remember also that melatonin and serotonin are not sedatives. But these two substances, derived from tryptophan, work together to help you sleep and wake consistently.

To eat better and sleep better, tryptophan is a must-have. It ensures a reliable production of serotonin and melatonin. Tryptophan is the least abundant amino acid in our food supply but it's still pretty easy to come by: There is more tryptophan in lamb, beef, and tuna than in turkey, and you'll find considerable quantities in plant-based foods such as nuts, seeds, beans, and whole grains. You can find a full list of sleep-supporting foods on page 70 so you can start stocking your kitchen with tryptophan-rich items.

Two Steps for Optimizing Your Tryptophan Intake

The *Eat Better, Sleep Better* plan is a straightforward one—but, it's not quite as simple as loading up your diet with tryptophan and calling it a day (and a sleep-filled night). Tryptophan alone won't increase your body's synthesis of melatonin and serotonin.

Why not? Because there are more plentiful amino acids in our food supply that can interfere with tryptophan's journey to the brain than there is tryptophan. In other words, tryptophan is outnumbered. The body is equipped with transport systems to shuttle compounds, including amino acids, in and out of cells, but these are shared systems. It's like a traffic jam in your body, and a caravan of 18-wheelers hauling competing amino acids, such as leucine or phenylalanine, are clogging the highways and boxing in your little compact car with its smaller load of tryptophan. Everyone is blocking your exit—the brain!

The road-hogging big rigs carting these other amino acids can delay, or even derail, the arrival of your modest shipment of tryptophan to the brain. (Remember, only 10 percent of the dietary tryptophan you consume is available for the brain, as most of it is absorbed into the bloodstream.) But, as with getting out of a traffic jam, there is a trick—and in a way it has to do with avoiding rush hour and trading up to a better vehicle. Here's a two-step solution to breaking that logjam and getting tryptophan where it needs to go, and it's all about what to eat—and when to eat it.

Step #1:
Combine protein and carbohydrates

If you eat tryptophan-rich proteins with carbohydrate-containing foods, such as legumes or whole grains, you'll trigger the release of insulin, the "traffic-cop" hormone that regulates blood sugar levels. Insulin goes to work, essentially directing all those other competing amino acids to flow more freely toward their respective cellular stops such as muscle and fat tissues, leaving less of them in the bloodstream. The insulin response effectively raises the relative proportion of tryptophan, figuratively clearing the road for tryptophan to board its transport system to the pineal gland located in the back of the brain, where the synthesis of melatonin and serotonin takes place.

Does this mean that you should have some cake after your steak? After all, the protein-rich beef contains tryptophan, and the cake is loaded with carbs. That is certainly not what I'm suggesting here. In fact, not all carbohydrates are equal, even if *all* carbs trigger the release of insulin. What you want are complex carbohydrates, which produce a more subtle insulin release. Refined carbohydrates, found in white flour and sugar (like the cake), trigger the insulin response, but not in a healthy way. Instead, they'll cause a sharp spike in your blood glucose levels, and that leads to a host of issues, including weight gain, increased risk for heart disease, and even cognitive issues such as brain fog, especially when you eat foods with refined sugar repeatedly and the glucose spike happens over and over.

Glucose, a simple form of sugar, is important—all your cells need it, including the brain and muscle cells. (The brain is especially dependent on glucose for energy and to function properly.) Insulin, in traffic-cop mode, directs glucose to be used as energy immediately or stored as glycogen, fuel for later.

In a healthy, active person with a balanced diet, the muscle cells use this reserve of glycogen for energy; when the glycogen runs out, the muscles burn fat. But when a person consumes more calories than they burn, particularly from refined carbs, a problem arises. When blood sugar levels rise in response to carbohydrate consumption and the muscle cells are already saturated with unused glycogen, they don't need or want another load of glucose, er, that cake. The extra sugar will eventually be converted to and stored as fat. (There are a number of

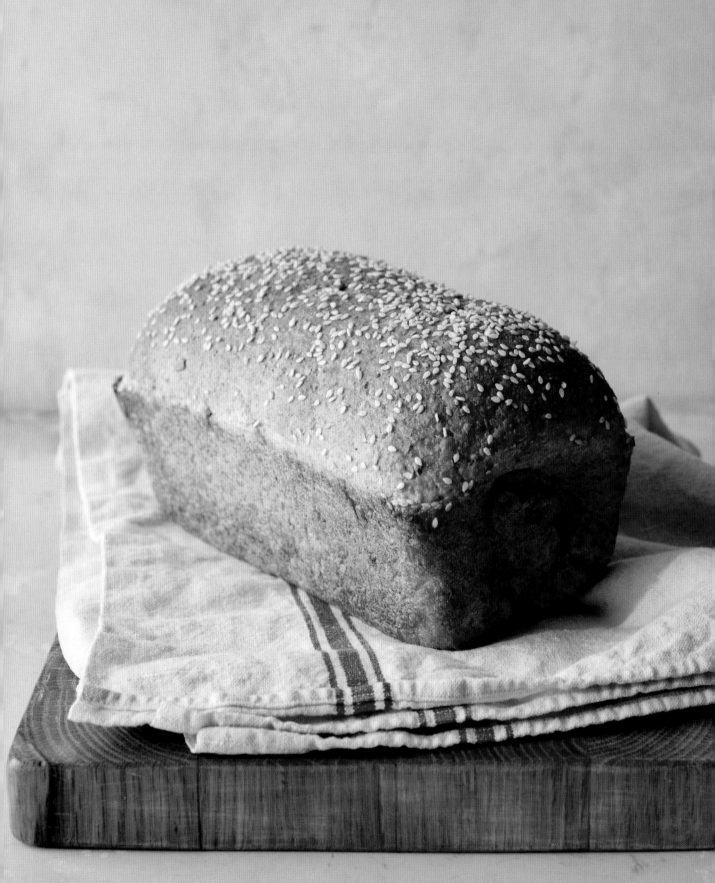

Sesame-Sunflower Oat Bread,
page 112

complex biochemical processes that cause this conversion, but fat storage is essentially the end result of too much glucose, or too much of anything, to be honest.)

High-carbohydrate intake overall also creates another issue: poor sleep quality. In our research, participants who consumed more refined carbs, including foods such as white bread and pasta, had more arousals, meaning they transitioned from deeper to lighter stages of sleep more frequently, throughout the night than others in the study.

How, then, do you combine protein with carbohydrates, so that you can get sleep-promoting tryptophan to the brain? The trick is to select carbs that won't send blood sugar levels on a roller-coaster ride of highs and lows. And this selection becomes more straightforward when you look for foods that deliver plenty of dietary fiber.

Choose fiber

As mentioned, *all* carbohydrates will cause the insulin response described above, but fiber-rich carbs will promote sleep—and won't spike your blood sugar, giving you that jolt of energy that a sugary slice of cake or cookie will. So, look for high-quality, nutritious carbs from minimally processed foods such as whole grains, beans, seeds, fruits, and vegetables. High-fiber foods move more slowly through your system, take longer for your body to break down and digest, and therefore keep your blood sugar levels on an even keel.

What you want to avoid are the refined carbohydrates in processed foods (like those salty pretzels or sugary cakes and cookies made from white flour) and foods such as white bread or crackers. These foods are high on the glycemic index, meaning that they can spike blood sugar, just the way sugar does. What's more, they lack nutrients and, most importantly, don't have the fiber you need as mentioned above.

If highly processed carb intakes are associated with less deep sleep, it follows that a slower rise in blood glucose, with more stable levels throughout the night, would create better conditions for the rejuvenating stages of our sleep cycles. My own research supports this premise. In a 2016 study, I found that participants who ate more fiber throughout the day had more deep sleep at night.

Step #2:
Eat sleep-supporting foods throughout the day

While it's key to know *what* to eat, it's just as important to know *when* to eat! The quick answer is "throughout the day"—and here's why that's true.

Nutrients from the foods we consume are not available to our bodies instantaneously. I'm not talking about what happens to your energy level when you drink coffee or an energy drink and eat a brownie, for example—those hits of caffeine and sugar generally work quickly on most people (and especially if you're sleep-deprived, beware the crash when the boost wears off). Instead, I'm referring to what takes place when you eat a full, well-balanced meal. It takes four to five hours for a meal to make its way through the stomach completely, and another two and a half to three hours for 50 percent of the small intestine to empty.

Proteins are broken down in the stomach and small intestine, and amino acids such as tryptophan are absorbed from the lower part of the small intestine. The journey of food through a healthy digestive system can take up to 40 hours (even longer for the elderly or those with constipation). This is why eating that tryptophan-loaded turkey sandwich or foods containing melatonin and serotonin such as dairy products, tart cherries, or tomatoes at 7:00 P.M. won't knock us out a few hours later.

Even if the normal digestive process was much speedier—imagine that load of tryptophan in your turkey passes your lips and takes the express elevator to your brain's pineal gland—your sleep mechanisms, including the production of melatonin, are still regulated by your personal circadian and homeostatic systems (see page 30). Melatonin production in the body is inhibited by light; its levels will rise in the evening, in response to darkness. You can't simply consume tryptophan to short-circuit such established responses in your body and sleep on demand.

Instead, eat sleep-supporting foods throughout the day, starting with breakfast, that will help you maintain a steady and available store of dietary tryptophan—there when you need it to facilitate serotonin synthesis and melatonin production. Working together, these compounds keep us alert in the morning and help us feel sleepy at night. The more regularly we consume the building blocks for the sleep response, the better for our bodies and brains. Think of it as keeping your pantry well stocked with staples—you don't want to run out of these essential ingredients, but with a bit of planning, you'll always have what you need.

Finding Foods That Will Put You to Sleep

Part 2 of *Eat Better, Sleep Better* is devoted to master lists of sleep-supporting ingredients, and Kat's delicious recipes, which anchor our eating plan. As you know by now, the way to ensure a steady supply of serotonin and melatonin is to combine protein-rich foods (for tryptophan) with fiber-rich carbohydrates (to optimize tryptophan uptake). We'll give you specific food lists as well as a 28-day eating plan that does just that, but the general information below will help you choose ingredients to put together your own sleep-supporting meals and snacks for a lifetime of healthy eating and sleeping.

First let's look at some big-picture guidelines—macro points on macronutrients, if you will, including choosing healthy carbohydrates, fats, and proteins. Then we'll take a quick look at some essential micronutrients for sleep. You'll also learn why it's generally better to get them from food (with some exceptions), rather than supplements.

Carbohydrates:
Choose foods with a low glycemic load

Any carbohydrate-rich food can trigger a tryptophan-motivating insulin spike, but as noted above, not all carbs are created equal, and those lacking healthy fiber are especially responsible for sending blood glucose levels soaring—and then crashing. You already know a frosted cupcake doesn't qualify as a whole-grain, healthy carb. But the sugar roller coaster can also be jump-started by some surprising sources.

No- or low-sugar foods such as white rice, pasta, that buttery fresh roll, and those low-fat pretzels will behave the same way in your system as that cupcake—even if they're organic and homemade. That's because white rice and white flour act just like sugar once they hit your system. The insulin traffic cop will treat them the same way it treats carbohydrates from a supersized soda. That's not to say that foods like pasta are off-limits, but it does mean that you should be aware of the glycemic load of the carbs you choose.

The glycemic index (GI) of a carbohydrate food is a numerical ranking system ranging from one to 100, designed to indicate how quickly that food will elevate your blood sugar level. Most professional charts developed by nutrition scientists will divide foods up as high (70 and above), medium (55–69), or low (less than 55). The higher the number, the faster the spike (and the worse for your insulin response). (High GI foods—even non-sweet foods that behave like sugar in the body such as white rice or crackers—are also linked to insomnia and other sleep disruptions. Eating a high glycemic index meal one hour before bedtime prolongs the time needed to fall asleep, compared to the same meal eaten four hours before bedtime.)

It can be a challenge finding a chart for everyday use and for non-professionals who don't work in healthcare or nutrition, as the data are often presented for medical or scientific use. You'll find a lot of information online about the glycemic index of different foods, but the most useful ones indicate a food's overall glycemic "load," which takes real-world serving sizes into account—and a food's weight and serving size matter. A white-flour hamburger bun can range from 30 grams for a small slider all the way up to 60 grams, which is a normal-sized bun. Investing in an inexpensive food scale can be worth it—and it's also a real eye-opener if you're concerned about portion control. The recipes and foods you'll find in *Eat Better, Sleep Better* are designed to be in the lower glycemic index range.

Also, though fiber-packed, nutrient-dense fruits are obviously a much better choice than a candy bar, be sure to look out for the GI of concentrated fruit sugars—processed dried fruits like banana chips or fruit "leathers" are considered high GI, as is fruit juice (which can deliver vitamins, but in a higher-calorie, no-fiber package, compared to whole fruit). Sweetened whole-grain breakfast cereals like granola can also creep into the higher ranges.

Fats:
Select sleep-supporting fatty acids

Just like carbohydrates, we know that not all fats are created equal. Healthy fats such as those found in nuts, avocados, tofu, eggs, chia seeds, and fatty fish like salmon provide important fat-soluble vitamins (A, D, E, K), and essential fatty acids—long-chain polyunsaturated fats that are particularly great for brain health and can lower rates of inflammation. And, not surprisingly, they are also associated with overall better sleep.

In 2016, my team published the results of an inpatient clinical intervention study of 26 healthy adults in the *Journal of Clinical Sleep*

Avoid High-Sugar Foods to Avoid This Condition

You may have heard the term *insulin resistance*. This refers to a breakdown of the insulin function—the insulin traffic cop is overwhelmed, likely from the consumption of dietary sugars from refined carbs and high glycemic foods and can't get all the glucose into the right cells. (There are also other reasons why people can become insulin resistant, but high-sugar foods are certainly involved.) The result is that glucose builds up in the bloodstream and this can have a devastating effect on your vascular system. Insulin resistance is serious and is a precursor to type 2 diabetes. But it can be controlled through early intervention, including diet and the avoidance of high GI and high glycemic load foods that cause large spikes in blood glucose.

Medicine that showed that eating more saturated fats—the fats found in ice cream, red meat, and just about every processed snack food and fast food—is associated with *lower* levels of deep sleep—the restorative healing sleep your body needs. In 2018, we published another study showing that eating a Mediterranean-style diet, which is well known to be low in saturated fats and higher in healthy fats from fish and olive oil, was associated with lower risk of insomnia and short sleep. There are also plant-based foods, including nuts and seeds, in a Mediterranean-style diet that provide sleep-promoting serotonin and melatonin.

One surefire way to incorporate these beneficial fats into your diet is to cook with them. Choose olive oil and other healthy plant-based oils, such as walnut, grapeseed and canola, and sunflower oil. Cold-pressed olive oil is excellent for salads and dressings, and extra-virgin olive oil, vegetable oil, and sunflower or soybean oil are best for medium-heat cooking; at high heat, extra-virgin olive oil degrades not only in flavor but also in nutritional value.

Plant-based oils are more heart-healthy than solid, highly saturated animal fats like butter and lard. (A good rule of thumb: Fats that stay liquid at room temperature are generally better for you than those that remain solid.) Besides good-quality oils, nuts, seeds, olives, avocados, fatty fish, and eggs, some dairy (including yogurt and milk) can be great sources of healthy sleep-supporting fats. As an added bonus, most of those foods contain inflammation-fighting antioxidants, such as the vitamin E found in foods like walnuts and the selenium in Brazil nuts.

Proteins:
Enjoy a variety of tryptophan sources

Though meat, poultry, and seafood are protein-rich foods that provide tryptophan, you can also look to plant-based proteins for it: For example, beans and legumes, nuts, seeds, tofu, and whole grains such as oats and brown rice are good sources of tryptophan.

A note on animal proteins: Most Americans get more than enough protein, but not necessarily good-quality protein, especially when it comes to meat. A double-bacon cheeseburger packs plenty of protein, but it's also delivering a load of saturated fat. And if you're eating protein from a fast-food source, you may also be consuming poor-quality, highly processed meat that is full of additives. And that's not also considering some of the accompanying refined carbohydrates.

Many people wonder exactly how much protein they need. It varies depending on body weight and activity levels, though active people don't need much more than sedentary people. (The daily recommendation is 0.8 gram per kilogram of body weight. For example, a 135-pound person—or 61 kilos—would need about 50 grams a day.) A healthy diet should contain at least 10 percent of calories from protein; for a 2,000-calorie diet, because there are 4 calories in a gram of protein, that's 50 grams. But most Americans are getting 15–17 percent of calories from protein, about 80 grams, so there is no need to supplement. The recipes in *Eat Better, Sleep Better* are designed to give you a healthy amount of quality protein from a variety of sources beyond meat.

Micronutrients for sleep

Beyond the proteins, carbohydrates, and fats that will support your tryptophan/serotonin/melatonin response, you need four essential micronutrients. Fortunately, these are widely available in the foods we've been discussing so far and in our eating plan. Here are the Big Four, along with some examples of sources for each. (You'll find a longer list of sleep-supporting foods on page 70–78.)

1. **ZINC:** Almonds, oysters, wheat bran

2. **MAGNESIUM:** Chia seeds, cashews, yogurt

3. **VITAMIN B$_6$:** Bananas, chickpeas, tuna

4. **FOLATE:** Broccoli, lentils, spinach

As you'll see in the tables provided on pages 70–78, some of these functional foods do double, triple, and even quadruple duty. Chickpeas, for instance, deliver all of the Big Four!

Should you supplement micronutrients?

You may be wondering if taking supplemental melatonin (as well as other nutrients, including those in our Big Four lineup) in the form of a pill, gummy, powder, or liquid, in addition to what you'll be getting from your diet, is a good idea. After all, you'd be contributing to your body's internal supply of this essential sleep ingredient, right? Why not just

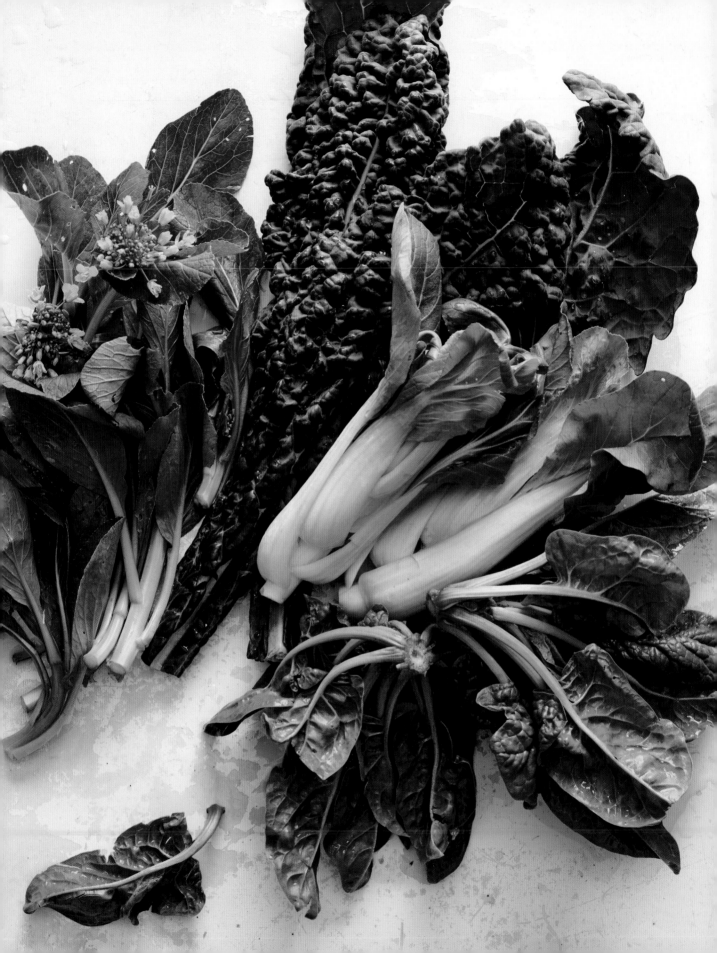

slip more into your system with an easy-to-swallow dose? Also, you've noticed these supplements are manufactured by reputable brands and sold in trusted stores. What's the downside?

Most supplements—and this applies to a wide swath of vitamins and minerals—you'll find in your drugstore or grocery store won't hurt you, unless you take excessive amounts beyond the recommended dosage or they interfere with medications you may be taking. But, they don't always help you and can end up being expensive. Even mass-produced supplements can be costly, and you may not be getting good quality or the most healthful form of a nutrient.

I always advocate eating food within a balanced diet as the best source of nutrients for most of us, and here's why: When it comes to nutrients, more is not always better, nor is it always effective to take isolated nutrients, which is essentially what a stand-alone supplement is. There's a famous study all undergraduate nutrition students learn about that illustrates these points, known as the ATBC study, short for alpha-tocopherol (vitamin E) and beta-carotene (vitamin A).

When researchers discovered that consuming more fruits and vegetables was associated with a reduced risk of cancer, they designed an interventional study to test causality. They enrolled white male smokers (at risk for cancer); one group took supplemental vitamin E, and the other group took vitamin A (vitamins found in fruits, vegetables, and vegetable oil). The ATBC study was stopped because there was more cancer in the beta-carotene group, while those taking alpha-tocopherol saw no benefits.

The take-home message from this study is this: Supplementing with excessive amounts of isolated nutrients—even if they are "good" for you—isn't always beneficial, and could in fact be harmful. Many nutrients have a sweet spot: Too little can mean a deficiency, but too much can also have adverse effects. In addition, consuming isolated nutrients can backfire. Take, for example, supplemental iron and calcium. These two substances compete for the same receptors in your cells, so too much of one prevents your body from absorbing the other effectively. This is why getting nutrients from a balanced diet is generally healthier and safer than supplements. Plus, absorbing nutrients from foods is more efficient than extracting them from supplements.

With food, you are taking in a combination of vitamins and minerals, and phytochemicals like polyphenols, that work together. Colorful fruits and veggies, which are rich sources of vitamins and minerals, come with plenty of other nonnutritive components, like polyphenols.

If you do take a multivitamin, here's why you should take it shortly after you wake up and not before bedtime: Some nutrients, like vitamin B_{12} and glutamine, have energizing effects that can disrupt sleep. But make sure to take them separately from your morning cup of coffee or tea, as caffeine reduces the body's ability to absorb iron and calcium. (For more information on caffeine, see page 58)

These polyphenols have important anti-inflammatory properties and can augment the health benefits of these foods beyond their micronutrient content. With a balanced diet, there is little risk of excess nutrients because in a healthy person, the body absorbs what it needs from food and excretes the rest.

That said, there are a few nutrients that are harder to get from food alone. Vitamin D, which our bodies make through exposure to sunlight, can be tough to get enough of if you're making it a point to stay out of the sun or if you live or work in an environment with little exposure to daylight. Getting enough iron can be a challenge if you don't eat meat or other animal products. If you don't consume dairy products, calcium may be an issue. (Some leafy greens like spinach contain calcium, but you'd have to consume 10 cups of raw spinach to get the same amount of calcium found in a cup of skim milk.)

High-quality supplements, including a good multivitamin, may be valuable, especially depending on your age and if you have specific health concerns. But don't self-diagnose and self-treat when it comes to supplements. Work with a licensed nutritionist or your health-care provider to make sure you're supplementing safely and that these supplements won't interfere with any medications you may be prescribed.

We have paid special attention to essential nutrients including calcium, vitamin D, and iron in putting together our eating plan because low amounts of these vitamins and minerals have been associated with sleep disorders, and they are often considered difficult nutrients to eat in sufficient quantities for some people. Our goal is to provide you with the information you need to get all the sleep-supporting nutrients you need through diet—and Kat's recipes are specifically designed to help you augment your melatonin and serotonin levels naturally, with great-tasting food.

What about melatonin supplements for sleep?

It's hard to ignore supplements marketed specifically for sleep, especially melatonin. It's everywhere. A popular nighttime cold remedy now touts melatonin as the main "natural" sleep ingredient. Transcontinental travelers have been buzzing about melatonin supplements for decades, swearing by its effectiveness in combating jet lag. Cheap supplements can be purchased at nearly any grocery or drugstore. But do they work?

The problem is that over-the-counter sleep-supporting supplements, including melatonin, "all-natural" herbal remedies, and CBD products are loosely regulated. As nonprescription products, they don't go through rigorous testing and scientific research, and their effectiveness and safety cannot be confirmed, despite what the marketing messages tell you. Some may even have unwanted side effects, like dizziness, headache, nausea, and day-after drowsiness. Some don't even contain the same amount of the ingredient as listed on the label.

As for popping supplements to sleep on the plane and avoid jet lag when you touch down at your destination, their effectiveness is mixed, and pales in comparison to a more reliable method for jet lag. Instead of crashing at your hotel after your 8:00 A.M. arrival and sleeping until the afternoon, try staying outside and getting some sunlight early in the day. Your circadian and homeostatic systems will get the message to reset more clearly from the sun than they will from a few melatonin capsules. (For a more detailed plan on circumventing jet lag, see page 55.)

While the two steps—what you eat and when you eat—that form the foundation of the *Eat Better, Sleep Better* plan are essential, healthy sleep habits are also important. Let's look at what constitutes healthy sleep, and what you can do—starting tonight—to get more of it.

Chapter 2

Eat Right to Sleep Right

My whole family keeps such regular hours when it comes to eating and sleeping that even our dog, Mojo, knows when it's time to head to bed. If we stay up past our usual bedtime on a weekend watching a movie, for example, Mojo leaves his spot on his cushion and goes to the back door for his nightly trip to the yard for a last potty before bedtime—and he's up at the same time in the morning, ready for his morning walk and breakfast.

Naturally, given my work, I'm attuned to the importance of regular sleep times when it comes to getting good-quality sleep, and the cardio-metabolic health benefits that come with it. Going to bed and waking up at the same time is an excellent habit if you want to sleep well, an idea that was ultimately included in the definition of sleep health, coined by Daniel J. Buysse, MD, distinguished professor of psychiatry, with an endowed chair in sleep medicine at the University of Pittsburgh and a leading figure in the world of sleep medicine.

Buysse reasoned that before we could treat sleep problems medically, we had to have a clear definition of the goal, which he proposed should be sleep health. Buysse initially suggested five measurable traits of a healthy baseline sleep pattern in individuals:

1. **SATISFACTION WITH SLEEP QUALITY**

2. **ALERTNESS DURING THE DAY**

3. **TIMING OF SLEEP**

4. **EFFICIENCY (HOW WELL YOU FALL AND STAY ASLEEP)**

5. **DURATION OF SLEEP (HOURS PER NIGHT)**

> It turns out that eating at regular intervals is also very important to both sleep and cardiometabolic health.

Buysse's sleep scale is a valuable tool in assessing sleep health. (See the quiz on page 50 to check your own sleep health.) Later, he added a sixth component that dovetails with my work: *regularity*, or regular sleep timing, meaning going to bed and waking up at the same time each day. It turns out that *eating at regular times* is also very important to both sleep and cardiometabolic health.

The Cost of a Lost Weekend

You work hard all week and keep a fairly regular meal and bedtime schedule, but come Friday night, you may go out for dinner, perhaps combined with a social event or entertainment. Instead of eating by 7:00 P.M., you're eating an hour (or maybe two) later, or you're munching on salty appetizers and sugary drinks and don't really get much of a meal. And even if you're not a social butterfly, you may still get a case of eating jet lag. Maybe you stay in and, because it's not a "school night," you eat a late dinner and then binge-watch your favorite show until 1:00 A.M. You sleep later the next morning. Perhaps you skip breakfast altogether and have a big brunch, then stay up and eat late again because . . . well, it's Saturday night. You sleep in on Sunday . . . and you see where this is going? Come Monday morning, it's hard to get going again—you've thrown off your circadian rhythms and your body is confused about the time of day. And by now, you're aware that can have a negative impact on your overall health.

Younger people between the ages of 18 and 25, like those in the Spanish study described above, may be more prone to this weekend roller-coaster pattern (if they lead a typical student or young professional life) and therefore may have higher levels of eating jet lag, but this irregular pattern can occur at any age. And as we age, our circadian rhythms are less robust, and it can take us a little longer to bounce back. That's why some of us might feel those late nights and late meals taking their toll on our brains and bodies a bit more as time goes on!

In 2017, on behalf of the American Heart Association (AHA), I chaired a committee that reviewed data on the importance of regular eating patterns—consistent meal timing and frequency—for cardiometabolic health. After reviewing extensive findings on the effects of irregular eating patterns on thousands of individuals (such as skipping breakfast, intermittent fasting, and fluctuations in the number of times one eats), the committee of scientists I led concluded that regular mealtimes boosted cardiometabolic health, while eating irregularities are associated with poor outcomes for heart health.[1]

More recent research from my lab shows that irregular eating is associated with higher levels of inflammatory markers in the body. And, eating meals later in the day is associated with weight gain. In a study of women, those who ate a greater proportion of calories after 8:00 P.M. and who did not eat a consistent amount on weekdays and the weekends gained weight and had an increase in waist circumference over a one-year follow-up period. One explanation for this could be because the body uses less fat for energy when you eat later at night.

---

1   On a related note, time-restricted eating and intermittent fasting have both been shown to have beneficial effects on cardiometabolic health stemming from weight loss. This weight loss can lead to better sleep, and fasting itself does not seem to have a negative impact on sleep. If you decide to try these techniques (with your doctor's approval), plan to break any fasts within two hours after waking for the day.

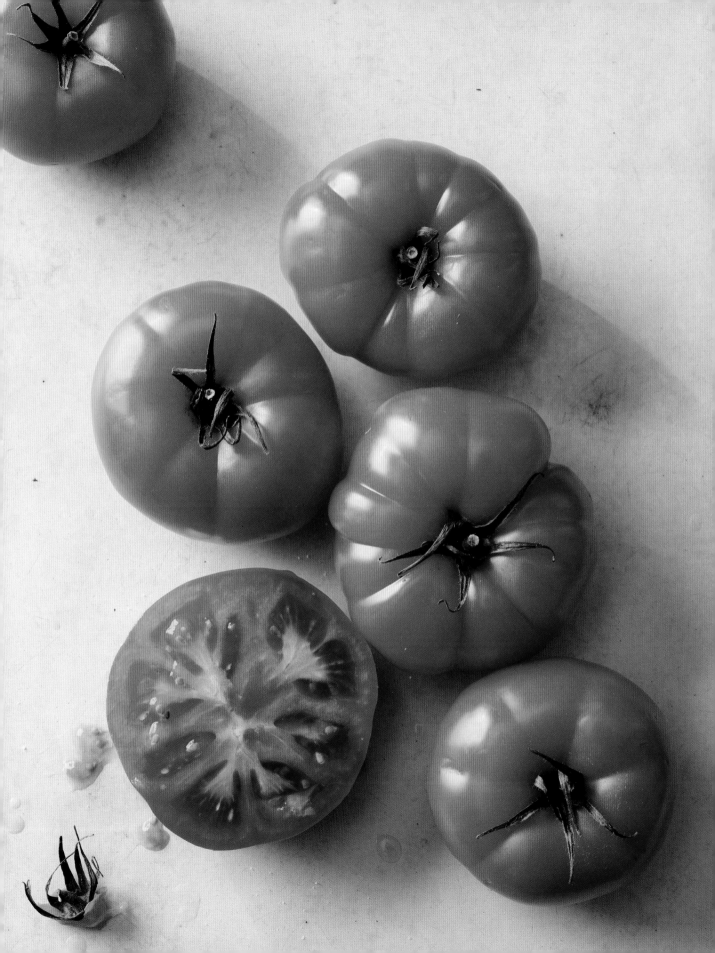

What does this have to do with sleep? Well, increased weight gain, poor blood pressure, and poor blood sugar control are all contributing factors to poor sleep.

Research my team and I conducted in 2020 showed a related finding. Those who stabilized their bedtimes lost weight and had lower levels of inflammation during a six-week study period compared to those who had variable bedtimes. We're following up on this idea with related research on the impact of regular rest and activity patterns. If you adopt a more regular sleep and activity/exercise schedule, will you have better blood sugar control and a healthier body weight? We're hoping to answer that question in one of my current studies. (And I think the answer will be yes.)

It's clear there are obvious health benefits to sticking with a regular eat-sleep schedule. If you take away one lesson in your quest to eat better and sleep better, it's this: Develop a routine and stick to it. Strive to eat nourishing meals at approximately the same time each day. And the same applies to sleep—try to be as regular in your habits as possible. That will also go a long way to helping you keep regular eating times!

Tackling Sleep Disorders and Disruptors

Sticking to a routine for eating and sleeping will help a lot, but you may still be facing some common sleep issues that plague many of us.

As mentioned earlier, Dr. Buysse's sleep quiz can be a handy way for you to self-assess your sleep health. R(u)SATED? That's the shorthand for the six markers of sleep health that make up his assessment.

Give yourself a 0 for rarely/never, 1 for sometimes, and 2 for usually/always. A score of 0 is considered poor sleep quality, while 12 is best. Once you calculate your score, you can start to address the individual issues to move yourself closer to a 12.

R IS FOR REGULARITY—Do you go to bed and wake up at the same time each day (within an hour)?

S IS FOR SATISFACTION—Are you satisfied with your sleep?

A IS FOR ALERTNESS—Do you stay awake all day without dozing?

T IS FOR TIMING—Are you asleep (or in bed) between 2:00 A.M. and 4:00 A.M.?

E IS FOR EFFICIENCY—Do you spend less than 30 minutes awake at night (including both the time it takes you to fall asleep and any awakenings in the night)?

D IS FOR DURATION—Do you sleep between six and eight hours every night?

How did you do? One way to improve your sleep, as you know by now, is to adopt the *Eat Better, Sleep Better* approach. But consistently good sleep can be elusive if you're battling a chronic sleep disorder like insomnia or sleep apnea, and I highly recommend you seek out treatment from your health-care provider (and let them know you're trying to address your issues through diet as well).

Understanding such conditions (discussed below)—and how diet can be used to address them—can help you hit the reset button. Fortunately, the dietary recommendations for each disorder are well-aligned with our *Eat Better, Sleep Better* eating plan.

Sleep disorders

INSOMNIA

Insomnia is a common sleep disorder characterized by difficulty falling and staying asleep, waking up too early in the morning, and feeling unrefreshed upon waking up. Insomnia can be acute; we all have our moments when our thoughts keep us from falling asleep at night. Maybe something happened at work or at home that you just can't shake out of your mind, or perhaps you fall asleep easily but wake up in the middle of the night or way too early and can't get back to sleep.

I've been there. One effective strategy I've borrowed from Aric Prather, PhD, professor of psychiatry at the University of California at San Francisco, is to get out of bed and write things down. I'm a big fan of making to-do lists, especially when I have a lot on my mind. It soothes me to plot out what I need to get done and allows me to let go of my thoughts and the fear of forgetting tasks. It's often that fear of forgetting that keeps us up, even more than the task itself. Plus planning out my time makes me see exactly how I can successfully take care of my to-do list on time, and that calms me down.

But sometimes insomnia can become chronic, meaning that those sleep perturbations mentioned above happen more than three times per

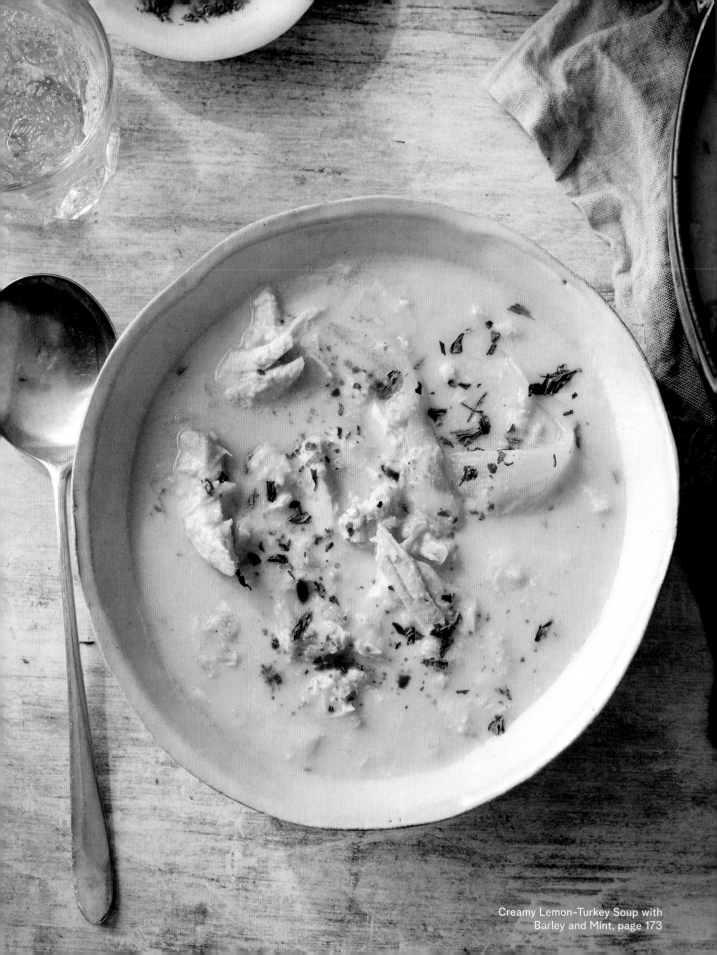

Creamy Lemon-Turkey Soup with
Barley and Mint, page 173

week for at least three months. The main course of treatment for this is cognitive behavioral therapy for insomnia, or CBT-i. Many psychologists are trained in this field and some apps can be helpful as well (see Resources, page 275).

Although what you eat won't *cure* insomnia, we know some foods contribute to this disorder. (There is plenty of research to bear this out, including the results of a 2020 population study that my team published in the *American Journal of Clinical Nutrition* that showed that women who ate a higher GI diet had increased rates of insomnia and were at a greater risk of developing insomnia in the near future.) Fortunately, we have also shown that certain diets can help manage and reduce the risk of developing insomnia, especially the well-researched Mediterranean diet, which features whole grains, an abundance of fresh fruits and vegetables, and healthy fats from olive oil and seafood rather than poultry and meat.

Our 2018 findings from the large medical research study known as MESA (short for Multi-Ethnic Study of Atherosclerosis), which includes nearly 7,000 Americans from diverse backgrounds, showed that middle-aged and older adults who ate a diet that aligned more closely with the Mediterranean diet had lower risk of insomnia symptoms, while those who reduced their adherence to this way of eating had a higher risk of developing insomnia symptoms over the subsequent ten years.

SLEEP APNEA

Obstructive sleep apnea (OSA) is a serious health condition that requires medical attention. This sleep disorder is one in which respiratory airways become blocked, resulting in loud snoring, breathing cessations, and sleep arousals (transitions from deeper to lighter sleep). When left untreated, sleep apnea can increase the risk of major cardiovascular problems, including coronary artery disease, arrhythmia, heart attack, and stroke. It's no wonder that the American Heart Association now recognizes sleep apnea as a risk factor for heart disease.

If you snore loudly or have a bed partner who has witnessed interruptions in your breathing at night (or maybe you notice this happening to your bed partner), please talk to your doctor about getting a sleep study. That will determine if you have sleep apnea and the best course of treatment.

An anti-inflammatory diet is associated with a reduced risk of OSA, according to a recent analysis from the National Health and Nutrition Examination Survey (NHANES). A six-month clinical trial in

180 overweight or obese patients with moderate to severe sleep apnea showed improvements in their symptoms with healthy lifestyle changes that included weight loss of 7 percent total body weight or more. If you have excess weight and are struggling with poor sleep due to OSA, slimming down and making other lifestyle changes, including incorporating a consistent eating and sleeping schedule, could be highly effective.

Our sleep-supporting approach to diet—rich in fiber, plenty of fresh fruits and vegetables, and a focus on lean protein and healthy fats—combined with light cardiovascular and resistance exercise, lines up with the AHA's recommendations for gradual and healthy weight reduction. Speak with your health-care provider before you embark on any weight-loss plan and consult a licensed nutritionist if you'd like additional help with your diet.

RESTLESS LEGS SYNDROME

As much as 10 percent of the U.S. population is affected by restless legs syndrome, or RLS (according to the National Institute of Neurological Disorders and Stroke), a neurological disorder characterized by leg discomfort and the irresistible urge to move the lower limbs. RLS symptoms tend to occur in the evening, which can make it difficult to fall asleep at night. The causes of RLS are not yet fully understood, but genetic predisposition and other environmental factors seem to play a role.

A meta-analysis of studies published in 2022 showed a connection between iron deficiency and RLS. In some people with a genetic predisposition for the disorder, iron deficiency seems to trigger symptoms, which can be reversed by consuming more iron. If your sleep is disrupted by RLS symptoms, have your iron levels tested. If you learn that you are iron deficient, you can work more iron-rich foods into your diet. Lean red meat (pork loin, lean ground beef, any cut of beef labeled "round" or "loin"), nuts and seeds, shellfish, and spinach are all great options. If you choose plant sources of iron, eating these foods with a good source of vitamin C will help with its absorption—for example, a flavorful spinach salad with clementine segments or strawberries (you can get even more by topping with sesame or pumpkin seeds). Calcium and caffeine reduce iron absorption, so be mindful of when you ingest those as well.

Depending on the severity of your iron deficiency and RLS symptoms, your health-care provider may also recommend supplements or other medications. Just be aware that iron deficiency is not the root cause of RLS for everyone. If your symptoms persist, consult your health-care provider.

Sleep disruptors

JET LAG

When we travel to a different time zone, jet lag inevitably sets in. This disorienting state is quite simply the abrupt misalignment of our body's two sleep-regulating systems: the homeostatic system, which dictates that sleep pressure builds up gradually over time awake, and the circadian system, which is regulated by natural daylight and darkness. But did you know that meal timing can be used to help you prepare for and rebound from jet lag?

Here's a neat trick: A few days ahead of traveling (or longer if you're traveling across more than a few time zones), start shifting your sleep, meal, and caffeine times gradually toward your destination's time, so your body's internal rhythms begin to align with the new location's clock. Make sure to expose yourself to morning sunlight once you arrive and be extravigilant about turning off bright lights and screens at night. This will help you to gently recalibrate your body's internal melatonin production and circadian rhythms.

When you arrive at your destination, start your days with a higher carbohydrate breakfast like our overnight oats (page 132) or smoothie bowl (page 136) to improve morning alertness. Exercise can help, too, particularly if you head outside in the morning for your preferred workout. You'll get the added benefit of natural bright light in the morning and an energizing jolt from the physical activity.

SHIFT WORK

Work that takes place outside of normal 9–5 business hours often goes by the shorthand of *shift work*, and it can interfere with the natural circadian and homeostatic systems for many workers—including those of doctors and nurses who are well aware of the negative impact that sleep disruptions have on health. Night shift work generally means a start time between 6:00 P.M. and 4:00 A.M., whereas early-morning shift work starts between 4:00 and 7:00 A.M., and afternoon/evening shift work starts between 2:00 and 6:00 P.M. Night shift work is frequently associated with sleepiness, reduced alertness and work productivity, and lower quality of life—to which Kat can attest from her years working as a professional bread baker.

Shift work disorder occurs when one cannot adapt to working at nonstandard times and experiences insomnia or excessive sleepiness with short sleep duration. These consequences of the work schedule occur for at least three months and are not better explained by another sleep disorder.

There are myriad adverse health effects associated with shift work, including increased risk of some cancers, obesity, cardiovascular disease, and type 2 diabetes. Pregnant evening shift workers also have a higher risk of gestational diabetes. There is currently high interest in the scientific community in uncovering strategies to help shift workers reduce their risk of chronic diseases. Frank Scheer, PhD, professor of medicine at Harvard Medical School, and his team have shown that eating during the daytime prevents glucose intolerance (when blood glucose stays high) and improves mood.

If you're working night shifts, it may not be convenient to eat *all* of your meals during the daytime, but you should consider making some changes to your usual mealtimes. A potential meal schedule for someone working midnight to 8:00 A.M., who is aiming to sleep six to seven hours when they get home, could include a complete meal late in the afternoon (e.g., 5:00 P.M.) and another meal around 8:00 P.M., a small mid-shift snack, and a light meal toward the end of the shift (e.g., 6:00–7:00 A.M.). If possible, avoiding bright light during the commute home in the morning (wear sunglasses when leaving your workplace) and exposing yourself to bright light in the evening will also help you sleep better during daytime hours and improve alertness at night. Make sure your bedroom is very dark and quiet for optimal daytime sleep.

Essentially, you're resetting your circadian and homeostatic systems—not easy to do, but worth the benefits for your sleep.

INDIGESTION AND ACID REFLUX

If your sleep suffers because of heartburn, you may be wary of a few common indigestion triggers in our recipes—most notably, tomatoes, alliums like onions and garlic, and peppers. Alliums and peppers are considered anti-inflammatory foods while tomatoes contain both serotonin and melatonin, so these ingredients can be useful in improving sleep health. Here are a few tips for enjoying the benefits of these foods while minimizing their triggering effects:

- When incorporating tomatoes into your diet, seek out lower acidity types, which include beefsteak, Roma, San Marzano, Campari, most yellow varieties, and any variety with *sweet* in its name.

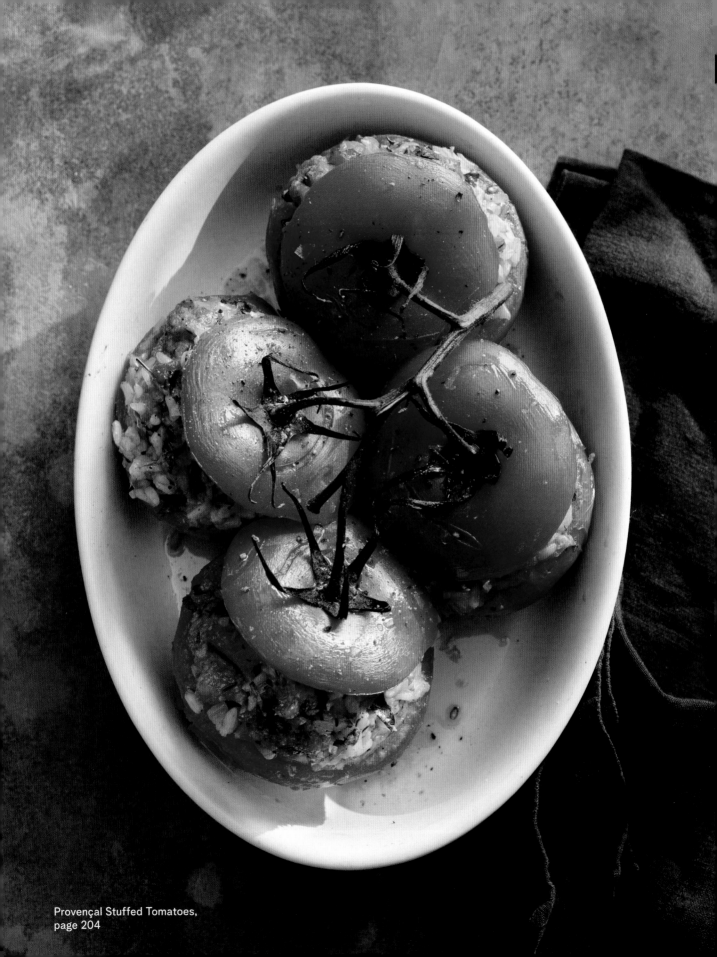

Provençal Stuffed Tomatoes,
page 204

- If you're especially sensitive to tomatoes, try removing their seeds before eating.

- After slicing or chopping onions, transfer to a sieve and rinse well under cold running water to remove some of their pungent, sulfurous compounds. Drain well before cooking or eating raw.

- Swap out "hotter" white or yellow onions with milder red or sweet varieties, shallots, or scallions.

- If alliums continue to trigger your symptoms, consider replacing them entirely with asafetida. Just a pinch of this spice (also known as hing), which is used widely in South India, provides a similarly pungent, oniony note without triggering acid reflux.

- Chiles often trigger heartburn; instead, opt for ginger in any form, or cinnamon. These spices bring robust flavor and warmth to dishes without the side effects of chiles. Plus, ginger, which also contains melatonin, has the added benefit of being a well-known home remedy for indigestion and nausea.

- Shift your consumption of irritating foods to earlier in the day and avoid eating them entirely for at least three hours before bed.

- Sleep with your upper body propped up with a pillow or cushion or sleep on your left side. The orientation of your organs will make it so that gravity works in your favor!

What about caffeine and alcohol?

Consuming certain dietary compounds can affect whether you're able to fall and *stay* asleep, and how much time you spend in the rejuvenating deep-sleep phase of your circadian cycle each night. Caffeine is an obvious offender, but here again, timing is key. If you're a coffee lover, you don't have to give it up. You do, however, have to pay attention to the clock.

My colleague Michael Grandner, PhD, associate professor of psychiatry and director of the Sleep and Health Research Program at the University of Arizona College of Medicine, says that most people don't use caffeine "appropriately." They drink it first thing in the morning and then often continue drinking it way too late in the day. Morning routines aside, we actually should wait an hour or two, after our first burst of waking energy wanes, before drinking our first cup of joe or tea. This way, we aren't interfering with our body's natural shift toward wakefulness by giving it a chemical assist from caffeine. I think this makes sense. (And intuitively, this is what I've always done because I don't like drinking coffee with multigrain cereal and skim milk, my go-to breakfast of choice!) A mid-morning cup of coffee tastes great and carries me to lunchtime. And then I'm done with coffee for the day.

Beware of the urge to drink caffeinated beverages in the afternoon. It takes about four to six hours for your body to metabolize and clear out just half the caffeine you ingest, so if you have a coffee drink or an iced tea at, say, 4:00 P.M., then go to bed at 10:00 P.M., half of that caffeine may still be having an effect. This is why you should avoid it in the hours before bedtime. This clearance also slows with age, so your cutoff point will shift earlier over time. Some people are extremely fast metabolizers when it comes to caffeine—those are the folks who can have an espresso after dinner and still fall asleep at 11:00 P.M. But for most of us, that's not the norm.

All that said, the best-loved sources of caffeine, including coffee, tea, and chocolate, contain heart-healthy polyphenols—compounds in plant foods like fruits and vegetables, which help reduce cellular damage and deterioration in the body—and even melatonin. Most people can safely enjoy the pleasures and health benefits of caffeine-containing beverages and foods in the morning, or by sticking with decaffeinated options after lunchtime. But, if you want to cut back or go entirely caffeine-free, I suggest doing so gradually. Some people experience severe withdrawal symptoms from stopping cold turkey.

I also suggest avoiding energy drinks and sodas entirely, both caffeinated and not, as they usually have little if any nutritional value, and their sugar content can disrupt sleep. Again, there are wide bodies of research, including my own, indicating that individuals who eat more sugar and other refined carbohydrates throughout the day have more sleep disruptions than people who have less sugar in their diet.

Now, what about unwinding at night with a drink? Unfortunately, alcohol—though it is a depressant and not a stimulant—can disrupt sleep cycles. The sedative effects of alcohol *can* help you get to sleep faster, but the quality of sleep that comes after a night of drinking is typically diminished, and regular overconsumption of alcohol can eventually result in sleep disturbances, a decrease in melatonin secretion and deep sleep, and even worsened obstructive sleep apnea.

If you do, however, enjoy wine or beer with your meal, you don't have to give them up for a good night's sleep. Rather, timing and moderation are key. Wine and beer both contain melatonin and other components that have been linked to overall health and well-being—including the well-known polyphenol resveratrol, a compound in red wine with anti-oxidant and anti-inflammatory properties. A glass with dinner shouldn't derail your circadian cycle, but I suggest not drinking alcohol, including hard liquor, for at least three hours before bedtime. If you'd like to reap the benefits of wine or beer without the boozy effects, consider incorporating these ingredients into your food instead; the alcohol will evaporate during the cooking process, leaving the flavors and beneficial components behind. (You'll find these ingredients used in some of our recipes.)

What to drink for sleep (and when to drink it)

In a word? Water. Adequate hydration is essential for healthy digestion, especially if you're active and eating a high-fiber diet, as fiber absorbs water. However, chugging a pint of water before bedtime isn't the best strategy. Your bladder's insistent wake-up call can be more unwelcome than the loudest alarm clock.

Aim for about eight cups of fluids per day, more if you live in a hot climate or if you're especially active and perspire a lot. (Coffee, tea, and juice also count as fluids, and raw fruits and vegetables are naturally packed with water.) If you're prone to waking up to use the bathroom during the night, front-load your hydration earlier in the day and aim to have your last glass with dinner, a few hours before bedtime. That said, don't go to sleep thirsty, either; a small glass of water or warm cup of herbal tea before bed is perfectly fine. As with caffeine, experiment with timing and see what works best for you.

What about warm milk? For generations, it's been a home remedy for insomnia and disrupted sleep, and while conclusive research into this specific beverage is limited, there is ample reason to believe there might be something to it. Milk contains tryptophan, melatonin, magnesium, and zinc, all of which support sleep. Couple that with the fact that a warm, non-caffeinated beverage can be a soothing way to wind down at the end of the day.

Another good option is to lightly sweeten warm milk with a teaspoon of honey or maple syrup to trigger a gentle insulin release that will help that tryptophan make its way into your brain. If you like to spice things up a bit, try also whisking in a quarter teaspoon each of soothing ground ginger and anti-inflammatory turmeric and a pinch of black pepper. This traditional Indian drink is known as haldi doodh, or golden milk, which has been recommended for sleep for generations. Avoid adding spirits; as I mentioned, alcohol tends to result in poor-quality sleep, especially close to bedtime—and it can also curdle milk!

Ages and Stages: How Sleep Changes Across Your Lifespan

As our bodies age and pass through different life stages, our nutritional needs and sleep health can change, too. My overall advice for a sleep-supporting diet can be applied at every life stage. However, understanding the science behind these changes arms us with the ability to adapt our diet and sleep for optimal sleep health at any age.

Teens

As anyone with a teenager might have noticed, their bedtime tends to get later and later starting in adolescence, peaking at around age 19. Their night-owl tendency will persist for a few years, but bedtime will generally start to shift back toward an earlier hour as they approach their mid-20s and adulthood sets in (along with increasingly adult responsibilities).

This late-night reset is caused by hormonal changes beginning in puberty, including a later time of melatonin release. (It's also reinforced by environmental factors, such as wanting to stay up late to watch TV or socialize, manage increasingly heavy school academic/athletic/social commitments, and more—including looking at their phones.) Adolescents and teens who go to bed later and later because they have a harder time falling asleep tend to sleep in late the next morning. I'm seeing this firsthand with my teenage twins, who can easily sleep in until 10:00 or 11:00 A.M. on weekends.

This is also why sleep and circadian rhythms researchers have been pushing for later high school start times: Early school days require students to wake up against their natural rhythm and can result in not getting enough sleep because of their tendency to go to bed late. This is problematic not only because growing bodies need sleep, but also because short sleep in teenagers is associated with learning difficulties, greater risk-taking behaviors such as reckless driving, and suicidal ideation.

Short sleep is associated with higher obesity risk (not just in adults, as previously mentioned, but in teens as well), and studies show that, when asked to cut their sleep short, teens tend to choose a higher GI diet marked by more added sugars, sugar-sweetened beverages and other carbohydrates, and fewer fruits and vegetables, setting in place the vicious cycle. When under-rested adolescents shift their eating to later at night, the foods they end up eating in the evening tend to be higher in fat and carbohydrates. These dietary behaviors go against all nutritional recommendations and are concerning as teens establish independent, lifelong eating habits. But they aren't surprising, either—these are the same food choices fatigued adults make when they need an energy spike.

So, parents, please resist that urge to get your teenager out of bed early on off days! They're not being lazy . . . they're just growing.

Pregnancy

Pregnant individuals are particularly susceptible to poor-quality and insufficient sleep for a variety of reasons, ranging from hormonal shifts to physical discomfort. Unfortunately, inadequate maternal sleep has been linked to poor maternal, fetal, and early childhood health. But there are ways to improve sleep quality for pregnancy, including the *Eat Better, Sleep Better* eating plan. If you are pregnant, talk to your health-care provider before you embark on any new diet plan.

We know that pregnant women who drink more sugary beverages tend to get less sleep—as is the case with nonpregnant people. Pregnant and breastfeeding mothers who followed the well-known DASH (Dietary Approaches to Stop Hypertension) diet (which tracks closely with the Mediterranean diet) reported taking less time to fall asleep, experiencing fewer sleep disorders, and having higher overall sleep efficiency. Infants of those mothers experienced fewer sleep disorders, too!

A 2021 study of pregnant women showed that those who stuck most closely to a Mediterranean diet—particularly one higher in olive oil— slept better, while those who ate more red meat tended to sleep worse.

For pregnant women with excess weight and obesity in particular, eating a diet higher in inflammatory foods such as refined carbs and processed meats is associated with taking a longer time to fall asleep, but conversely, eating an anti-inflammatory diet can be beneficial.

As I mentioned earlier, limiting refined sugars and red meat while favoring a lower GI diet rich in olive oil, fish, low-fat dairy, and minimally processed plant foods is good advice for anyone looking to improve their sleep. If you're pregnant, these dietary choices may be even more important.

Sleep and the aging adult

The circadian system that ensures we sleep, eat, and wake at the right time weakens with age. It provides less resistance against the homeostatic system (which builds sleepiness during the day) and doesn't work as well during the night. The end result? We start to fall asleep a bit earlier and wake up earlier as well, once that sleep pressure has been dispensed.

This is because as we age, our internal melatonin production starts to wane, though the extent of this decline varies from person to person. Unsurprisingly, those who have greater reductions in melatonin levels experience more trouble sleeping. These people also tend to have other health concerns such as inflammatory disorders, heart disease, and hypertension—all of which also negatively impact sleep. These factors can kick off the dreaded vicious cycle, this time implicating melatonin: Aging people with health concerns have greater declines in melatonin, which negatively impacts their ability to get refreshing sleep, leading to further declines in health.

For women, a diet low in salt and sugar and higher in lean protein, minimally processed carbs, and fiber during menopause is linked to better sleep. However, associations between diet and sleep are frequently found to be at their most prominent in the years leading up to and during menopause, due to related hormonal fluctuations that impact serotonin levels.

There is ample research to support a significant sleep-food connection even later in life, for both men and women. A recent study that looked into diet and risk of sleep apnea in nearly 146,000 nurses and health professionals showed stronger associations between diet and sleep apnea risk in adults over the age of 65. In 2019, my team published a study that showed a lower risk of insomnia in postmenopausal women who ate a lower GI diet rich in fruits, vegetables, and fiber, and an increased risk of insomnia in women eating more added sugars and refined grains. Others have also found similar associations in men. Collectively, research shows that even small dietary changes can make a big difference in our sleep quality and overall health as we age.

Resetting Your Sleep Cycle

Whether you're battling a chronic sleep disorder, dealing with one of the external sleep disruptors mentioned in this chapter, or having trouble sleeping for other reasons, focusing on breaking the harmful cycle of poor sleep on overall cardiometabolic health is the first step toward better sleep health. The food lists and recommendations, our 28-day eating plan, and the recipes that follow in the next part of this book will help you sustain healthy sleep.

Here are a few daytime and nighttime tips for getting and staying on track—but you don't have to wait to totally reset your sleep cycle before you start eating more healthily, the *Eat Better, Sleep Better* way.

DAYTIME:

- **Eat a healthy breakfast.** The data are consistent: Breakfast skippers have worse-quality sleep than breakfast eaters, perhaps because breakfast eaters are maintaining and reinforcing strong circadian rhythms. Growing up, I would wake to a glass of freshly squeezed orange juice that my mom would serve my sister and me to drink alongside our breakfast cereal, always a vast selection of low-sugar, whole-grain options. (I still love my cereal and don't restrict myself to eating it only for breakfast, and there are good options out there beyond the junky sugar-loaded types marketed to kids.) Breakfast consumption has been associated with better sleep at night and we provide many good options in this book. You may not like to eat first thing in the morning, but your metabolism and blood sugar levels will benefit if you eat within two hours of waking up, and you're reinforcing healthy circadian rhythms.

- **Be physically active.** Any physical activity—ideally outside and during the daytime to expose yourself to natural light—is helpful for sleep because you are supporting your body's natural circadian rhythms. Avoid strenuous activity too close to bedtime. Scientists haven't yet identified the perfect combination for sleep health, but I favor calmer activities like yoga and tai chi in the evening and more intensive cardiovascular workouts earlier in the day, as vigorous exercise increases your alertness and raises body temperature, making it harder to fall asleep. But the bottom line is this: Any activity is good for sleep, so if your choices are not exercising at all or exercising in the evening (because that's the only time you can do so), then I'd say exercise. Just make sure to slow your activity afterward, take a warm shower, and dim the lights.

- **Limit daytime naps.** If you are too sleepy to maintain wakefulness during the day, a quick power nap may be the solution. Just make sure to do this early, before 4:00 P.M., and keep it short—30 minutes or less. Why early? Because you want enough time after this nap to build back some sleep pressure to feel sleepy at the appropriate time at night. Why short? Because you don't want to relieve your full sleep drive. In other words, save some of your "sleep pressure" so that it's still easy for you to fall asleep quickly at night. (Note: 4:00 P.M. may be too late if you go to bed early, say 9:00 P.M. If you choose to nap, give yourself at least six hours between naptime and bedtime.)

NIGHTTIME:

- **Wind down before bedtime and stay away from devices and bright light.** Not only will they contribute to stress (just think of reading that demanding or unpleasant email just before you go to bed), but they'll prevent your natural melatonin levels from rising, making it harder to ease into sleep.

- **Sleep in a cool, dark, and quiet environment.** Blackout curtains can be a great investment to provide a dark room and they can also help reduce outside noise.

- **Remove stimulants and sleep disruptors like caffeinated drinks, alcohol, nicotine, and heavy meals close to bedtime.** Maybe you have a pet who is restless and noisy at night or insists on sleeping with you in a way that's comfortable for them, but less than ideal for you (cats and dogs have a gift for doing just that); give them their own space so that you can have undisturbed sleep. Although our dog, Mojo, would love to sleep with us, my husband and I insist he stay in his own room for the night, complete with a baby gate to make sure he doesn't find his way to our bedroom door.

- **Keep consistent bedtimes.** My work has shown that women who stabilize their bedtime have reductions in body fat mass. In a six-week period, women who adopted consistent bedtimes reduced their weight by 1.5 pounds.

Part 2

Eat Better to Sleep Better: The Plan

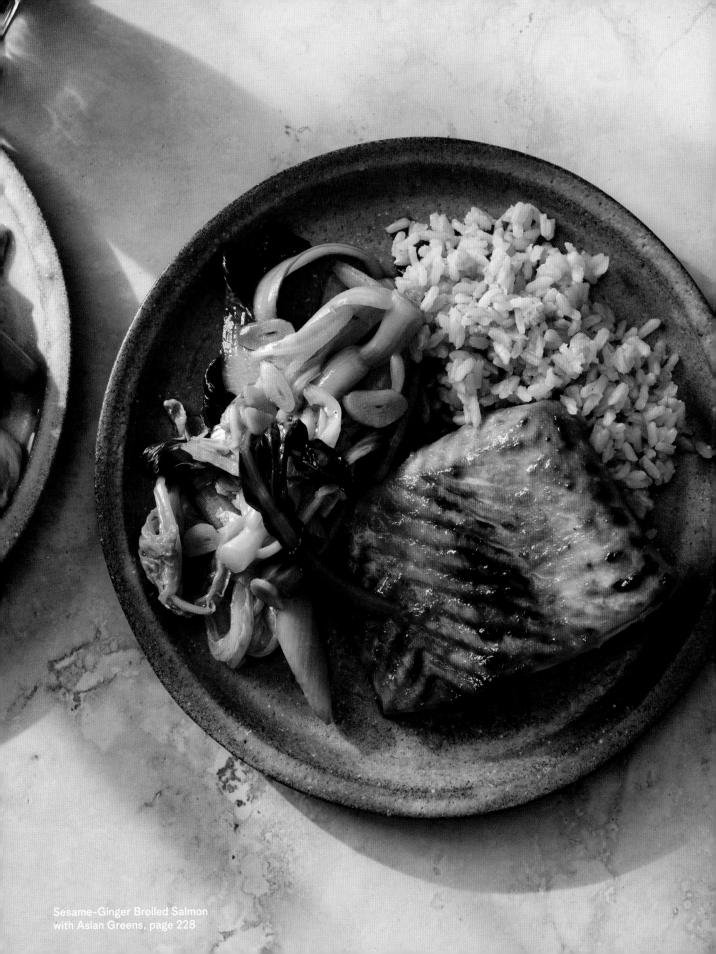

Sesame-Ginger Broiled Salmon
with Asian Greens, page 228

Chapter 3

Food for Sleep

Even small tweaks to your diet can improve your sleep quality almost immediately. In a study my team published in 2016, we found differences in "sleep architecture"—the different stages of sleep such as light and deep sleep—on *the same day* that participants changed their diets. There are myriad factors, including age, general health, and current sleep patterns, that contribute to how quickly sleep will get better, but all studies show that even the slightest changes to diet improve sleep.

Everyone is different. But I'm confident that four weeks of making the right food choices—or just sticking with our plan to take the guesswork out of those choices—will result in falling asleep faster and achieving better-quality sleep and the many other health benefits that come with it.

About the *Eat Better, Sleep Better* Eating Plan

Our 28-day plan, which you'll find on pages 85–88, provides you with three sleep-supporting meals a day, ensuring that you'll consume an assortment of foods with nutrients that are necessary for efficient melatonin and serotonin synthesis in the brain.

You'll see some elements of the heart-healthy Mediterranean diet—foods high in unsaturated fats such as olive oil, seafood, nuts, seeds, legumes, fruits and vegetables, and whole grains. But we go well beyond the traditional Mediterranean diet to incorporate a range of foods that will boost your body's sleep mechanisms—protein sources like turkey, shrimp, and tofu; carbohydrates such as buckwheat and oats; and a variety of flavors and spices including ginger, cumin, and turmeric. In fact, we used my own findings and incorporated components of four well-known approaches to healthy eating, all associated with improved sleep. In addition to the Mediterranean diet, we incorporated tenets of a low-sodium diet, an anti-inflammatory diet, and a low glycemic index diet.

The resulting *Eat Better, Sleep Better* diet is a delicious eating plan low in saturated fat, sugar, and sodium, and high in fiber, micronutrients, and phytochemicals. This is an approach to food that you can embrace for a lifetime, and you'll enjoy numerous health benefits besides improved sleep quality.

Eat Better, Sleep Better Master List of Sleep-Supporting Ingredients

The tables in this section include foods with sleep-supporting components. You can use this information to diversify your regular diet and to modify our recipes to your own tastes and dietary needs. The ingredients in the first two lists are rich in dietary tryptophan and the four essential nutrients linked to serotonin and melatonin synthesis. The second two lists contain ingredients with natural melatonin or serotonin.

Tryptophan-Rich Ingredients

Tryptophan is an amino acid that can be found in both animal- and plant-based protein sources. When consumed alongside healthy carbohydrates, it can kickstart our body's internal production of melatonin and serotonin, both of which are important for regulating the circadian cycle. **The minimum dietary recommendation for tryptophan is 250 milligrams per day,** but to produce improvements to sleep health, we suggest choosing protein sources that are higher in tryptophan whenever possible.

LEGUMES	MG PER SERVING	SERVING SIZE
Edamame	97	½ cup (cooked)
Lentils	80	½ cup (cooked)
Tofu	155	½ cup
White beans	102	½ cup (cooked)

MEAT AND DAIRY	MG PER SERVING	SERVING SIZE
Beef	294	3 oz.
Chicken breast	307	3 oz.
Clams	288	3 oz.
Egg	77	1 large
Lamb	282	3 oz.
Pork	292	3 oz.
Salmon	211	3 oz.
Tuna	243	3 oz.
Turkey	248	3 oz.
Yogurt (low-fat)	51	6 oz.
Yogurt (nonfat)	54	6 oz.

NUTS, SEEDS, AND GRAINS	MG PER SERVING	SERVING SIZE
Almonds	60	1 oz.
Barley	91	1 cup (cooked)
Brown rice	219	1 cup (cooked)
Buckwheat groats	76	1 cup (cooked)
Cashews	81	1 oz.
Chia seeds	87	2 Tbsp.
Flaxseed	84	1 oz.
Multigrain bread	35	1 oz.
Oats	74	½ cup (cooked)
Peanuts	71	1 oz.
Pistachios	71	1 oz.
Pumpkin seeds	168	¼ cup
Sesame seeds	124	¼ cup
Sunflower seeds	122	¼ cup
Walnuts	48	1 oz.

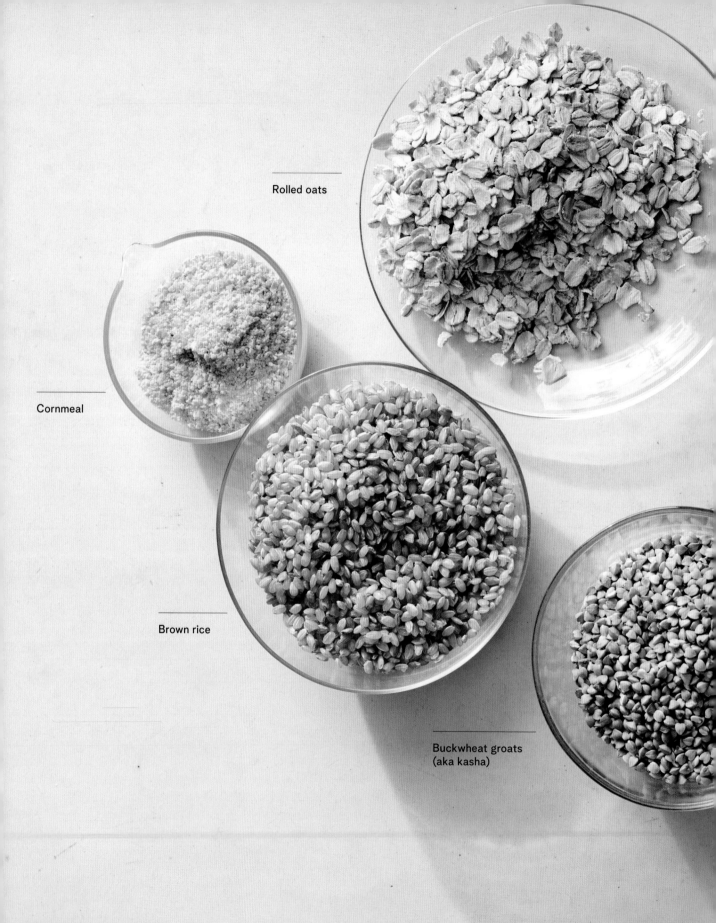

Rolled oats

Cornmeal

Brown rice

Buckwheat groats
(aka kasha)

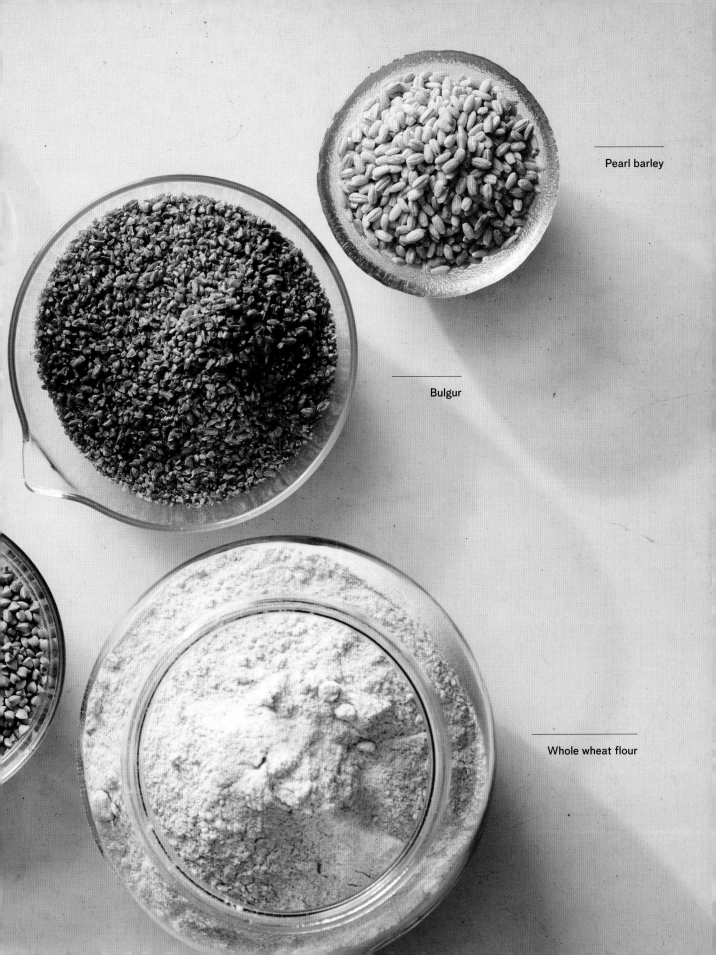

Pearl barley

Bulgur

Whole wheat flour

Additional Sleep-Enhancing Nutrients

Vitamin B$_6$, folate, zinc, and **magnesium** are particularly important for supporting our body's production of serotonin and melatonin. A daily serving of any of the following ingredients is a good or excellent source of at least one of these four important nutrient boosters—and sometimes all of them.

INGREDIENT	RICH IN
Almonds	Magnesium, zinc
Banana	B$_6$, magnesium
Beets	Folate, magnesium
Broccoli	Folate, B$_6$
Cashews	Magnesium, zinc
Chickpeas	Folate, B$_6$, magnesium, zinc
Collard greens	Folate, B$_6$, magnesium
Lentils	Folate, B$_6$, zinc
Mango	Folate, B$_6$
Marmite	Folate
Oysters	B$_6$, magnesium, zinc
Pumpkin seeds	Magnesium, zinc
Rapini	Folate, B$_6$
Spinach	Folate, magnesium
Tofu	Magnesium, zinc
Wheat bran	Folate, B$_6$, magnesium, zinc

Serotonin-Rich Ingredients

In humans, serotonin is produced in the gut as well as the brain stem, where it helps regulate body temperature, mood, behavior, attention, sleep, and wakefulness. It has also been detected in certain plants. **Eating these foods (all of which are also rich in micronutrients, antioxidants, and other anti-inflammatory compounds) supports our own internal serotonin and melatonin production.**

INGREDIENT

Avocado	Green pepper	Orange	Plantain	Strawberry
Banana	Hazelnuts	Papaya	Plums	Tomatoes
Bok choy	Kiwi	Passion fruit	Scallion	Walnuts
Chicory	Lettuce	Pecans	Spinach	Wild rice
Chocolate	Nettle	Pineapple		

Melatonin-Rich Ingredients

Eating foods rich in melatonin helps to support our own melatonin production, thereby regulating a healthy sleep cycle. Animals produce melatonin for the same reasons humans do—to help regulate their circadian cycles. But melatonin can also be found in plants; the highest levels tend to be concentrated in the plants' reproductive organs, particularly the seeds.

FRUITS AND VEGETABLES

Apple	Onions
Banana	Oranges
Cabbage	Pepper
Cranberry	Pineapple
Cucumber	Pomegranate
Garlic	Purslane
Goji berry	Radishes
Grapes	Rainier cherries
Kiwi	Strawberries
Mango	Tart cherries
Mushrooms	Tomatoes

ANIMAL PRODUCTS

Beef

Cheese

Chicken

Egg

Lamb

Milk

Pork

Rainbow trout

Salmon

Sea bass

Yogurt

PANTRY

Almonds	Fennel seed	Sunflower oil
Anise seeds	Flaxseed	Sunflower seeds
Balsamic vinegar	Ginger	Tart cherries
Barley	Grapeseed oil	Tomatoes
Beer (particularly dark)	Kidney beans	Turmeric
Cardamom	Lentils	Walnut oil
Celery seeds	Mustard seeds	Whole wheat flour
Coffee	Oats	Wine (particularly red)
Coriander seeds	Pistachios	
Cornmeal	Rice (particularly brown, black, and red varieties)	
Extra-virgin olive oil	Soybean oil	

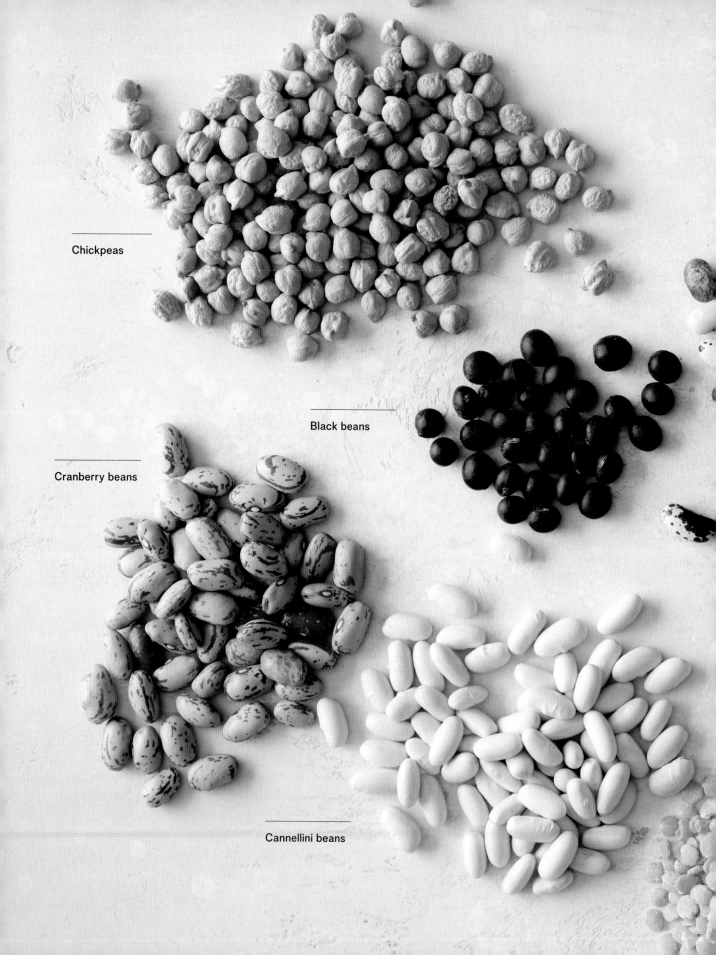

Chickpeas

Black beans

Cranberry beans

Cannellini beans

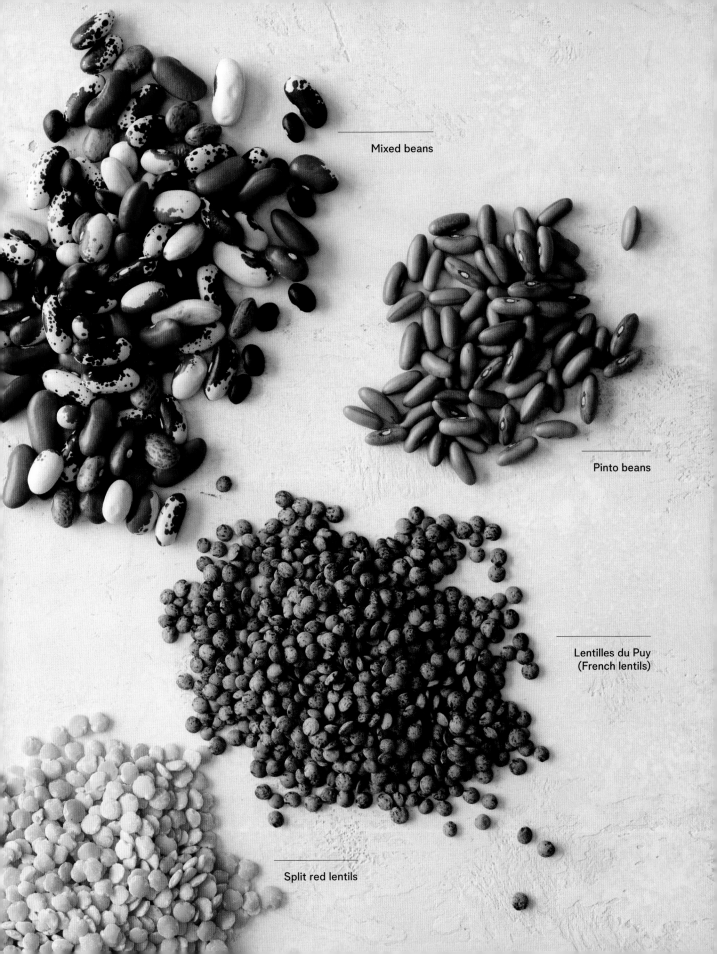

Mixed beans

Pinto beans

Lentilles du Puy
(French lentils)

Split red lentils

My Top 20:
Powerhouse Ingredients to Stock Your Sleep-Supporting Kitchen

FOOD	SLEEP-SUPPORTING COMPOUNDS
Almonds	Tryptophan, fiber, melatonin, magnesium, omega-6 fatty acid, zinc
Bananas	Fiber, complex carbohydrates, serotonin, melatonin, magnesium, vitamin B_6
Barley	Tryptophan, fiber, complex carbohydrates, melatonin, magnesium, vitamin B_6, zinc
Brown rice	Tryptophan, fiber, complex carbohydrates, melatonin, vitamin B_6, magnesium, zinc
Cherries	Fiber, complex carbohydrates, melatonin
Chia seeds	Tryptophan, magnesium, omega-3 and omega-6 fatty acids, fiber, complex carbohydrates, vitamin B_6, zinc
Extra-virgin olive oil	Melatonin, monounsaturated fatty acids, polyphenols
Ginger	Melatonin, polyphenols
Lentils	Tryptophan, fiber, melatonin, magnesium, zinc, vitamin B_6, folate
Oats	Tryptophan, fiber, complex carbohydrates, magnesium, zinc
Pineapple	Fiber, complex carbohydrates, serotonin, melatonin
Pumpkin seeds	Tryptophan, fiber, magnesium, zinc
Salmon	Tryptophan, melatonin, omega-3 fatty acids, vitamin B_6, vitamin D, vitamin B_{12}
Spinach	Fiber, folate
Tofu	Tryptophan, magnesium, zinc
Tomatoes	Fiber, complex carbohydrates, melatonin, vitamin B_6
Turkey	Tryptophan, vitamin B_6, magnesium, zinc
Walnuts	Tryptophan, serotonin, melatonin, omega-3 and omega-6 fatty acids, vitamin B_6, magnesium, zinc, fiber
White beans	Tryptophan, fiber, folate, magnesium, zinc
Yogurt	Tryptophan, melatonin, zinc, probiotic, vitamin B_{12}

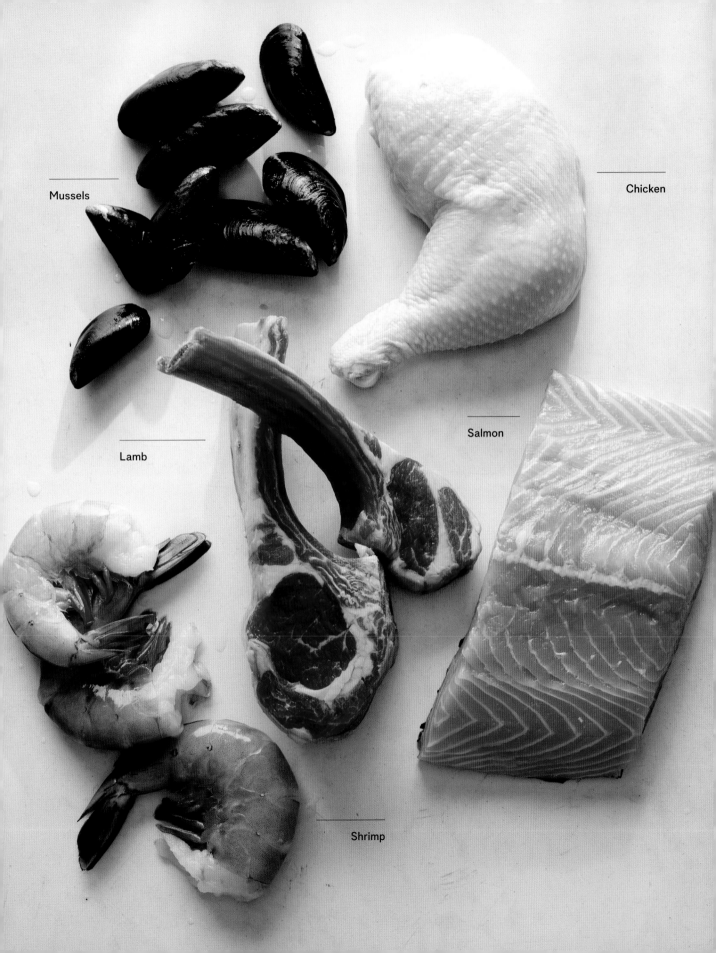

Mussels

Chicken

Lamb

Salmon

Shrimp

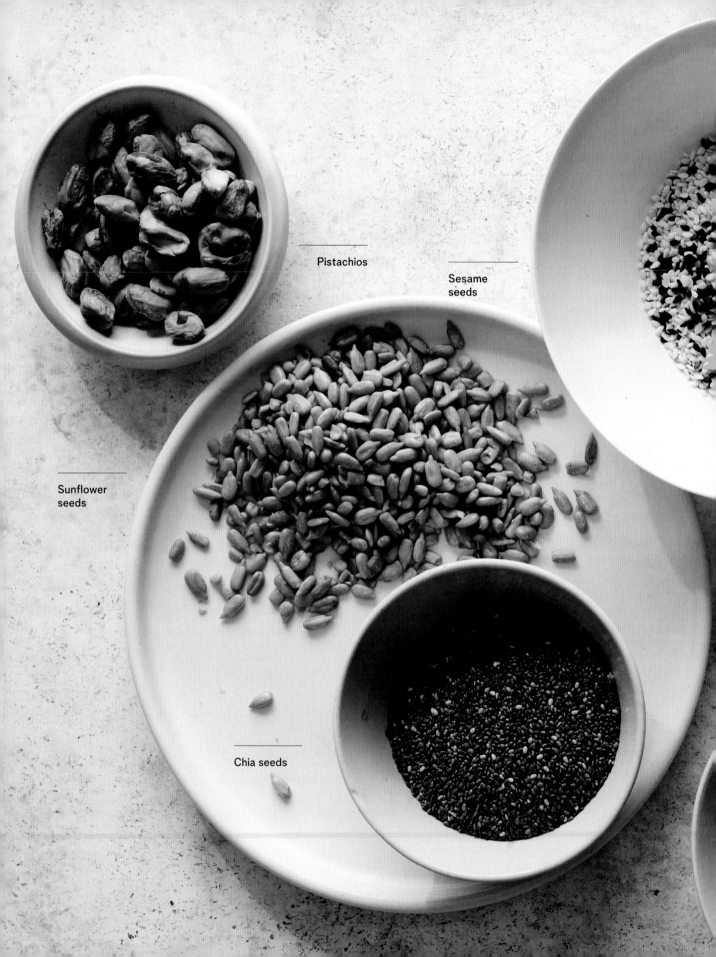

Pistachios

Sesame
seeds

Sunflower
seeds

Chia seeds

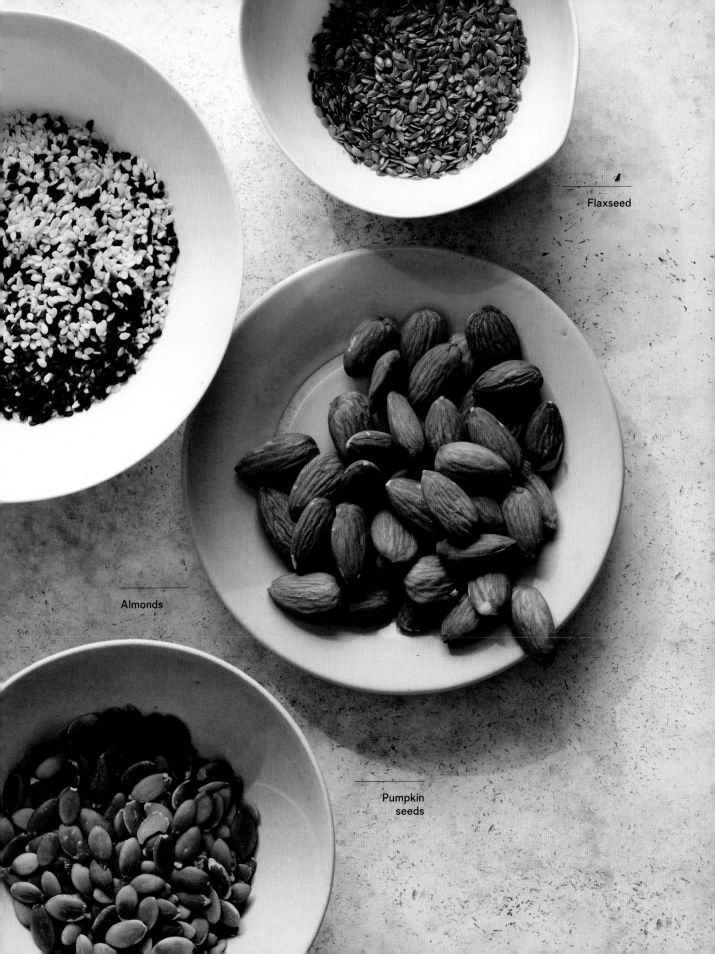

Flaxseed

Almonds

Pumpkin
seeds

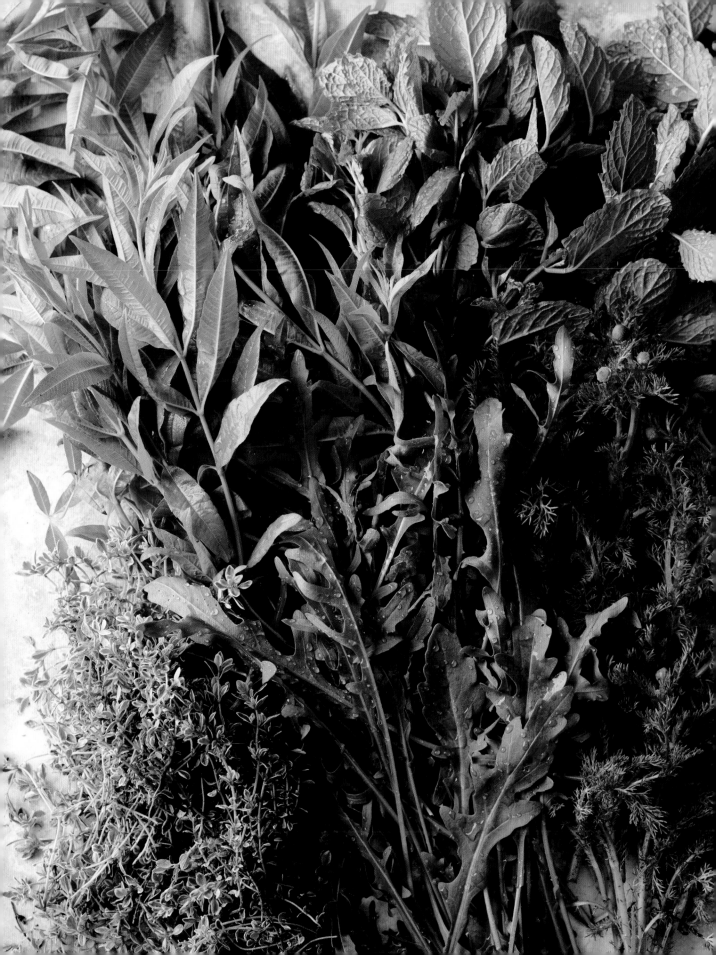

LOWERING YOUR FOOD COSTS—TIPS FOR REDUCING WASTE AND SAVING MONEY:

- **Buy in bulk when you can:** We use ingredients such as whole grains, nuts, and seeds frequently throughout this book. Buying in bulk saves money as well as packaging. Store nuts and seeds in airtight containers or zip-top freezer bags in the freezer.

- **Make swaps:** Although our recipes lean into plants and plant-based ingredients, we do include a moderate amount of animal and fish protein, too. Feel free to swap out similar items based on cost, availability, and sustainability. For example, the price of fresh fish fluctuates significantly and can be particularly pricey away from the coasts. If fresh options are limited, don't overlook the freezer section. If you have a local butcher or fishmonger, talk to them about what you're making and what is most affordable or on sale.

- **Shop wisely for produce:**

  Organic fruits and vegetables are a plus, but they aren't associated with better sleep.

  Shop seasonally whenever possible. In-season fruits and vegetables are fresher and more nutritious, sustainable, and more affordable than items that have been shipped from the other side of the world. Delicate fruits like berries and stone fruit are at their cheapest and most delicious in the summertime.

  Fill your freezer with peak-season ingredients so you have them ready to use throughout the colder months. To retain their freshness, wash and dry berries, pitted cherries, or other small fruits, then spread them out on a large rimmed baking sheet and transfer to the freezer. Once they're frozen solid, transfer to airtight containers or zip-top freezer bags and store in the freezer for up to six months.

- **Stock up on herbs and spices:** We love these natural flavor enhancers. Many herbs and spices have proven sleep-supporting effects and others just taste great. These can be pricey at conventional grocery stores, so instead, stock up on these pantry staples at spice shops; online (you'll find some of our favorite online sources on page 275); or Asian, Middle Eastern, or South American markets. Their spices are typically fresher than anywhere else and often less expensive, too, because they are buying in bulk and moving inventory so quickly.

- **Grow what you can:** If you have the space to do so, consider growing your own fresh produce. Seed catalogs and local nurseries offer a staggering range of options for some of our favorite sleep-supporting ingredients like heirloom tomatoes and leafy greens. And your kids will love eating all of the greens from your (and their) garden. Even apartment-dwellers can flex their green thumbs—with a little love, many fresh herbs will thrive in a sunny indoor spot.

- **Shop at farmers' markets when possible:** The freshest ingredients and least processed foods come directly from those who grow and make them. Many farmers' markets now accept government-sponsored nutritional assistance benefits, formerly known as food stamps. To find out if you are eligible, contact your local SNAP (Supplemental Nutrition Assistance Program) office.

Four Weeks to Better Sleep

This meal plan is designed to take the guesswork out of what to eat to improve your sleep. Each day is nutritionally balanced to provide all the vitamins, minerals, and other compounds you need to optimize your body's internal melatonin production. If you stock your pantry, freezer, and fridge with the ingredients on pages 70–78, you will have taken the first step to getting in the habit of cooking and eating for better sleep health.

WEEK ONE	DAY 1	DAY 2	DAY 3	DAY 4	DAY 5	DAY 6	LAZY WEEKEND
Breakfast	Banana-Berry Smoothie Bowl with Chia and Granola (p. 136)	Overnight Oats with Ginger, Winter Compote, and Walnuts (p. 132)	Maple-Pecan Muesli (p. 131)	The Restful Smoothie (p. 268)	Spiced Buckwheat Porridge with Dates, Tahini, and Greek Yogurt (p. 135)	Savory Whole Wheat Dutch Baby with Turkey Bacon, Kale, Tomato Butter, and Eggs (p. 151)	Muffin-Tin Quiche with Salmon, Goat Cheese, and Spinach (p. 138)
			Plain yogurt	Make-Ahead Morning Muffins (p. 150)			Little Gem Salad, Blue Cheese Buttermilk, Tomatoes, and Garlic Croutons (p. 170)
Lunch	Barley Salad with Spinach, Feta, Pickled Mushrooms, and Walnuts (p. 174)	Fresh green salad, tinned fish or chickpeas, Creamy Sesame-Ginger Vinaigrette (p. 115)	Chilled Out Soba Salad with Edamame and Sesame-Ginger Vinaigrette (p. 165)	Creamy Lemon-Turkey Soup with Barley and Mint (p. 173)	Spiced Red Lentils with Coconut, Sweet Potato, and Greens (p. 181)	Cold Marinated Tofu with Sesame and Scallions (p. 198)	
	Tuscan White Bean Dip (p. 107), crudités	Make-Ahead Morning Muffins (p. 150)	Fresh kiwi	Seeded Cornmeal Crackers (p. 108), cheese	Whole wheat naan or pita	Brown rice	Beet Hummus (p. 105), crudités
Dinner	Pan-Seared Halibut with Barley-Artichoke Risotto (p. 222)	Spiced Red Lentils with Coconut, Sweet Potato, and Greens (p. 181)	Smoky Oyster Chowder with Saffron, Fennel, and Kale (p. 177)	Sesame-Ginger Broiled Salmon with Asian Greens (p. 228)	Lamb Stew with Bulgur, Almonds, Dried Fruit, and Fresh Herbs (p. 209)	Green Spring Gumbo with Chicken Andouille (p. 212)	Provençal Stuffed Tomatoes (p. 204)
	Fresh kiwi	Brown rice	Crusty whole-grain bread	Sesame Shortbread Cookies (p. 237)	Roasted Figs with Walnuts and Greek Yogurt (p. 243)	Chamomile-Ginger Panna Cotta with Midsummer Compote and Pistachios (p. 259)	Crusty whole-grain bread
		Sesame Shortbread Cookies (p. 237)	Sesame Shortbread Cookies (p. 237)				Maple-Pumpkin Crème Caramel (p. 241)

WEEK TWO	DAY 8	DAY 9	DAY 10	DAY 11	DAY 12	DAY 13	LAZY WEEKEND
Breakfast	Buckwheat Crepes with Apple-Walnut Filling (p. 235)	Sleep-Better Egg Toast with Goat Cheese, Lemon, and Greens (p. 144)	Granola (p. 146–147)	Whole Grain Chicken Porridge with Scallions and Sesame-Cashew Crunch (p. 216)	In-a-Hurry Egg-and-Cheese with Salsa Roja (p. 143)	Whole Wheat Pancakes, Tropical Fruit Compote, and Sesame-Cashew Crunch (p. 160)	
			Sliced banana				
			Plain yogurt				
Lunch	Warm Pita Salad with Kale, Feta, Tomatoes, and Chickpeas (p. 166)	Tomato Salad with Anchovy, Green Olives, and Onions (p. 169)	Fresh green salad, tinned fish or chickpeas, Creamy Sesame-Ginger Vinaigrette (p. 115)	Muffin-Tin Quiche with Salmon, Goat Cheese, and Spinach (p. 138)	Garlic Shrimp with Nori Butter and Lemon (p. 231)	Fresh green salad, Creamy Sesame-Ginger Vinaigrette (p. 115)	Family Brunch: Dry-Marinated Skirt Steak with Fried Eggs, Pickled Mushrooms, and Grilled Tomatoes (p. 156)
	Beet Hummus (p. 105), crudités	Crusty whole-grain bread	Plantain Cake with Yogurt–Cream Cheese Frosting (p. 246)	Fresh green salad, Creamy Sesame-Ginger Vinaigrette (p. 115)	Fresh green salad, Creamy Sesame-Ginger Vinaigrette (p. 115)	Plantain Cake with Yogurt–Cream Cheese Frosting (p. 246)	Creamy Tahini Cocoa (p. 271)
					Crusty whole-grain bread		
Dinner	Chickpea Gemelli with Butternut Squash, Walnuts, and Parmesan (p. 194)	Whole Grain Chicken Porridge with Scallions and Sesame-Cashew Crunch (p. 216)	Garlic Shrimp with Nori Butter and Lemon (p. 231)	Mushroom "Carbonara" with Broccoli Rabe and Parmesan (p. 189)	Grilled Chicken Cutlets with Midsummer Mostarda (p. 207)	Turkey and Black Bean Burrito Bowl with Salsa Verde (p. 219)	Portuguese-Style Tomato Rice with Mussels and Scallops (p. 203)
	Oven-roasted broccoli, Garlicky Fish Sauce Dressing (p. 127)	Plantain Cake with Yogurt–Cream Cheese Frosting (p. 246)	Fresh green salad, Creamy Sesame-Ginger Vinaigrette (p. 115)	Oven-roasted butternut squash		Banana-Chamomile Shortcake (p. 252)	Winter Compote (p. 100)
	Midsummer Compote (p. 98), frozen yogurt		Brown rice				Sesame Shortbread Cookies (p. 237)

WEEK THREE	DAY 15	DAY 16	DAY 17	DAY 18	DAY 19	DAY 20	LAZY WEEKEND
Breakfast	Granola (p. 146–147)	The Restful Smoothie (p. 268)	Overnight Oats with Ginger, Winter Compote, and Walnuts (p. 132)	Make-Ahead Morning Muffins (p. 150)	Maple-Pecan Muesli (p. 131)	Sweet Whole Wheat Dutch Baby with Honey-Butter Bananas, Greek Yogurt, and Almonds (p. 155)	Muffin-Tin Quiche with Salmon, Goat Cheese, and Spinach (p. 138)
	Plain yogurt			Banana	Plain yogurt		Fresh green salad, Creamy Sesame-Ginger Vinaigrette (p. 115)
	Banana			Almond butter	Blueberries		
Lunch	Turkey and Black Bean Burrito Bowl with Salsa Verde (p. 219)	Spiced Red Lentils with Coconut, Sweet Potato, and Greens (p. 181)	Little Gem Salad, Blue Cheese Buttermilk, Tomatoes, and Garlic Croutons (p. 170)	Barley Salad with Spinach, Feta, Pickled Mushrooms, and Walnuts (p. 174)	Spiced Red Lentils with Coconut, Sweet Potato, and Greens (p. 181)	Tomato Salad with Anchovy, Green Olives, and Onions (p. 169)	Seeded Cornmeal Crackers (p. 108)
	Fresh green salad, Creamy Sesame-Ginger Vinaigrette (p. 115)	Seeded Cornmeal Crackers (p. 108)	Plain yogurt	Orange	Sesame-Sunflower Oat Bread (p. 112)	Sesame-Sunflower Oat Bread (p. 112)	Cheese
			Kiwi			Tuscan White Bean Dip (p. 107)	
Dinner	Smoky Oyster Chowder with Saffron, Fennel, and Kale (p. 177)	Lemony Baked Trout (p. 220)	Chilled Out Soba Salad with Edamame and Sesame-Ginger Vinaigrette (p. 165)	Savory Chickpea Pancake with Shrimp, Saffron, and Arugula (p. 227)	Sopes with Black Beans, Queso Fresco, and Curtido (p. 183)	Sesame-Ginger Broiled Salmon with Asian Greens (p. 228)	Pan-Seared Halibut with Barley-Artichoke Risotto (p. 222)
	Focaccia with Beefsteak Tomatoes and Olives (p. 187)	Spiced Carrots and Parsnips with Tahini-Lemon Sauce (p. 197)	Chia Pudding with Tropical Fruit Compote and Greek Yogurt (p. 249)	Tropical Fruit Compote (p. 101), frozen yogurt or sorbet	Banana-Chamomile Shortcake (p. 252)	Soy-Braised Butternut Squash with Miso Butter and Black Sesame (p. 193)	Oven-roasted Brussels sprouts, Garlicky Fish Sauce Dressing (p. 127)
	Apple sauce, Sesame-Cashew Crunch (p. 104)	Easy Stone Fruit Sorbet (p. 250)				Brown Rice Pudding with Saffron, Dates, and Pistachios (p. 256)	Blackberry-Plum Galette with a Corn Crust (p. 253)

WEEK FOUR	DAY 22	DAY 23	DAY 24	DAY 25	DAY 26	DAY 27	LAZY WEEKEND
Breakfast	The Restful Smoothie (p. 268)	Brown Rice Pudding with Saffron, Dates, and Pistachios (p. 256)	Overnight Oats with Ginger, Winter Compote, and Walnuts (p. 132)	Granola (p. 146–147)	Sleep-Better Egg Toast with Goat Cheese, Lemon, and Greens (p. 144)	Make-Ahead Morning Muffins (p. 150)	Buckwheat Crepes with Apple-Walnut Filling (p. 235)
	Make-Ahead Morning Muffins (p. 150)	Sliced banana		Midsummer Compote (p. 98)		Creamy Tahini Cocoa (p. 271)	
				Plain yogurt			
Lunch	Muffin-Tin Quiche with Salmon, Goat Cheese, and Spinach (p. 138)	Turkey sandwich with lettuce and tomato on Sesame-Sunflower Oat Bread (p. 112)	Cold Marinated Tofu with Sesame and Scallions (p. 198)	Fresh green salad, tinned fish or chickpeas, Creamy Sesame-Ginger Vinaigrette (p. 115)	Spiced Red Lentils with Coconut, Sweet Potato, and Greens (p. 181)	In-a-Hurry Egg-and-Cheese with Salsa Roja (p. 143)	Little Gem Salad, Blue Cheese Buttermilk, Tomatoes, and Garlic Croutons (p. 170)
	Fresh green salad with Creamy Sesame-Ginger Vinaigrette (p. 115)	Midsummer Compote (p. 98)	Fresh green salad with Creamy Sesame-Ginger Vinaigrette (p. 115)	Plantain Cake with Yogurt–Cream Cheese Frosting (p. 246)	Sesame-Sunflower Oat Bread (p. 112)		Focaccia with Beefsteak Tomatoes and Olives (p. 187)
		Plain yogurt					Cheese
Dinner	Warm Pita Salad with Kale, Feta, Tomatoes, and Chickpeas (p. 166)	Pan-Seared Halibut with Barley-Artichoke Risotto (p. 222)	Spiced Red Lentils with Coconut, Sweet Potato, and Greens (p. 181)	Portuguese-Style Tomato Rice with Mussels and Scallops (p. 203)	Provençal Stuffed Tomatoes (p. 204)	Lemony Baked Trout (p. 220)	Grilled Chicken Cutlets with Midsummer Mostarda (p. 207)
	Tuscan White Bean Dip (p. 107), crudités	Oven-roasted kale, Garlicky Fish Sauce Dressing (p. 127)	Seeded Cornmeal Crackers (p. 108)	Sesame Shortbread Cookies (p. 237)	Seeded Cornmeal Crackers (p. 108) with cheese	Soy-Braised Butternut Squash with Miso Butter and Black Sesame (p. 193)	Chia Pudding with Tropical Fruit Compote and Greek Yogurt (p. 249)
		Plantain Cake with Yogurt–Cream Cheese Frosting (p. 246)	Blackberry-Plum Galette with a Corn Crust (p. 253)			Roasted Figs with Walnuts and Greek Yogurt (p. 243)	

ANYTIME SNACKS

Tuscan White Bean Dip (p. 107) or Beet Hummus (p. 105), crudités

Sesame Shortbread Cookies (p. 237)

Granola (p.146–147) or Sesame-Cashew Crunch (p. 104), plain yogurt

Fruit Compote (p. 98–101), plain yogurt

Opposite: Maple-Pumpkin Crème Caramel, page 241

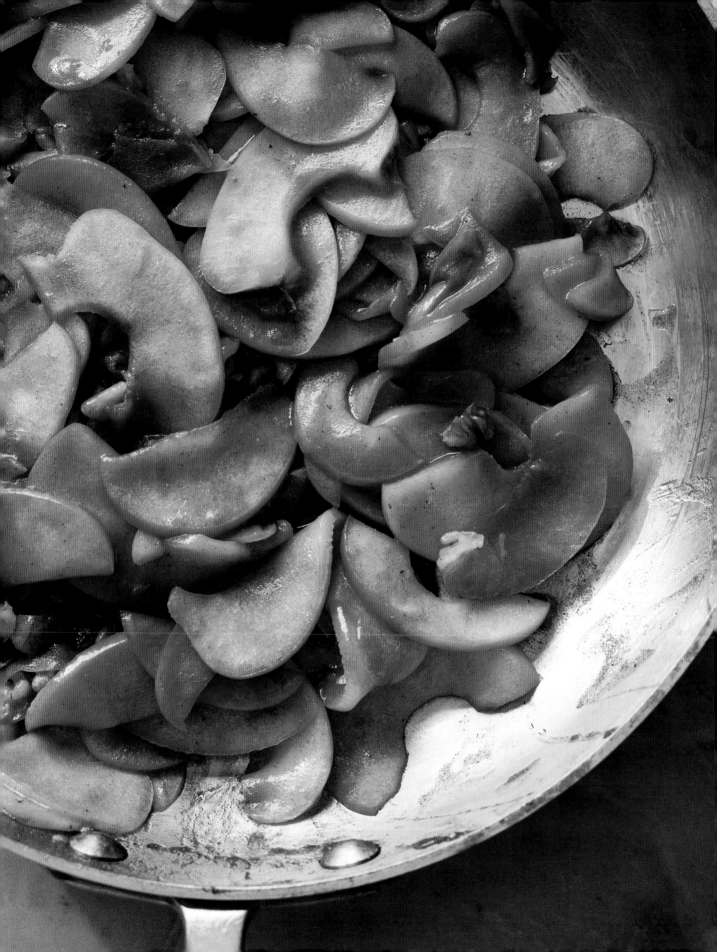

Chapter 5

Eat Better to Sleep Better: The Recipes

Having worked in the food business for many years— first in high-pressure restaurant kitchens, and then in the cookbook and food magazine business—I've been fortunate when it comes to sleep. The physical demands and rush of kitchen work and a varied diet blessed me with many years of deep, blissful, and largely uninterrupted sleep.

Then COVID-19 hit. Like so many others, I quickly pivoted to working from home. Holed up in my New York City apartment, I spent a lot more time sitting at my laptop—and a lot less time walking and exercising. In general my day-to-day food choices became more monotonous. I took fewer trips to the supermarket, meaning my diet—usually rich in fresh fruit, vegetables, and seafood—started to skew toward the pantry and its bounty of white rice, sugars, and pastas. Add to that a bit more white wine than usual and more late-night screen time and you can bet I found myself regularly watching the clock tick toward dawn.

In late 2020, when Marie-Pierre and I started talking about her research, I was a little suspicious—how could a few extra salads and salmon fillets influence how I was sleeping at night? But the more she walked me through study after study showing clear connections between diet and sleep, the more the science started to make sense. We decided that together, we would use her findings to develop a book of easy, crowd-pleasing, *sleep-supporting* recipes.

The following chapters are loaded with these nutritionally balanced, easily adaptable dishes, all designed to promote healthy sleep. Ease your way in with one or two—my favorites are the Portuguese-Style Tomato Rice with Mussels and Scallops (page 203) and the Sesame Shortbread Cookies (page 237), and Marie-Pierre is partial to the Cocoa Nib Granola with Candied Ginger, Cherries, and Almonds (page 147), the Soy-Braised Butternut Squash with Miso Butter and Black Sesame (page 193), and the Savory Chickpea Pancake with Shrimp, Saffron, and Arugula (page 227). Then, when you're ready to get on the fast track to better sleep, dive into the meal plan (page 85). These sleep-supporting meals are a pleasurable and effective path toward better sleep at any age.

—Kat Craddock

Getting Started

The recipes are designed for usability

Our goal is to make it easy for you to incorporate foods throughout the day that will result in a good night's sleep. Most of the dishes come together quickly, and throughout the recipe chapters, we've provided meal prep ideas to make them even easier to assemble after a busy day. We've also included a handful of slightly more involved recipes perfect for a leisurely weekend. Trust that these more time-consuming dishes call for very little active prep—we don't expect you to spend every weekend cooking, after all.

Depending on your usual diet, you may notice that our recipes call for more ingredients than you're used to; this is intentional. The best, most well-balanced (and most interesting!) diets are rich in micronutrients from a variety of sources. We recommend buying plenty of shelf-stable ingredients like whole grains, seeds, nuts, legumes, dried fruit, and extra-virgin olive oil in bulk because these foods turn up repeatedly throughout our recipes. Check out our shopping guide on page 275 for a few of our favorite online sources. (And remember: Nuts and seeds should be stored in the freezer to maintain their freshness.)

A note on yields, nutrition, and cook times

The yields and cook times listed throughout are approximations—we all chop onions at our own pace and we all have different caloric needs. While this book was not designed with weight loss in mind, you might find that you lose weight with our recipes and 28-day plan. That's because the recipes are generally high in fiber from an abundance of fresh produce and whole grains, and they have been formulated with an eye to the USDA and American Heart Association's guidelines for a generally healthy balance of fats, complex carbohydrates, lean plant- and animal-based proteins, and essential, sleep-supporting micronutrients.

It's likely other metabolic health markers including blood pressure, glucose, and lipid profile will improve as well. If you *don't* want to lose weight, consider the included recipe yields and meal plan to be suggestions—very active adults and growing teenagers may consume a larger portion than what we've suggested, and that's okay! Eat slowly, pay attention to your own body's needs, and stay hydrated. If you feel you need further direction on how much you should be eating, consult with your health-care provider or a nutritionist. Finally, you may already be eating a variety of independently healthy ingredients, but combining them in the right way—as Marie-Pierre's studies show—is key to promoting better sleep; the recipes are designed to bring ingredients that work together, together.

Season to taste

Takeout, restaurant food, and processed foods are often loaded with added salt and sugar, so generally, once we start cooking at home using raw ingredients, our sugar and salt consumption tends to drop. Many of the recipes in this book eschew set salt measurements and instead ask the cook "season to taste." We really mean that! Taste your food as you cook and add salt (a little bit at a time—once it's in there, you can't take it out!) until the dish tastes good to you.

Dairy direction

Dairy products such as milk, cheese, and yogurt are excellent sources of dietary tryptophan. Whole-milk versions of these foods are, however, high in saturated fat. The American Heart Association recommends that adults and kids go with fat-free or low-fat options, and Marie-Pierre's own research shows that a diet higher in saturated fat is associated with less overall deep sleep. Unless otherwise specified, the recipes in this book calling for milk and yogurt were developed using fat-free versions, and we believe they're perfectly delicious that way.

Most other fat-free cheeses and butter substitutes, however, tend to be highly processed and contain fillers, sugars, and stabilizers that adversely affect their texture and flavor. When using butter and most cheeses, we chose quality over quantity; in other words, use the real stuff—in careful moderation.

Stock the pantry

Before you dive in, we suggest stocking your kitchen with the foods and ingredients in tables on pages 70–78 because they'll be used frequently throughout the rest of the book. Whether you're a novice or experienced cook, it's always more motivating to make something if you know that you have most of the ingredients on hand before getting started. Additionally, having a handful of these items prepped ahead of time (such as cooked grains) makes it easier to sneak in an extra dose or two of flavor and sleep-supporting goodness on the fly. (But don't worry—if you're eager to get something on the table *tonight*, all of our make-ahead pantry items can be quickly substituted with store-bought equivalents; you'll find plenty of specific recommendations to that effect wherever they're needed.)

Food Allergies and Sensitivities

If you suspect that you have a food allergy, an allergist can help you determine which foods to avoid. Food sensitivities, which tend to be less severe, are much tougher to diagnose, but an elimination diet can help you identify common intolerances. Once you know which foods are a problem for you, the next steps are between you and your health-care provider. If your reactions are mild and you choose to still eat these problematic ingredients, we suggest limiting them to the earlier half of the day to be sure your body has a chance to process and recover from any reactions by bedtime.

The recipes in this book can be adapted to accommodate most common food allergies and sensitivities. Keep an eye on the headnotes and sidebars for substitution suggestions throughout and bookmark our Master List of Sleep-Supporting Ingredients (see page 70) for additional, tasty swaps.

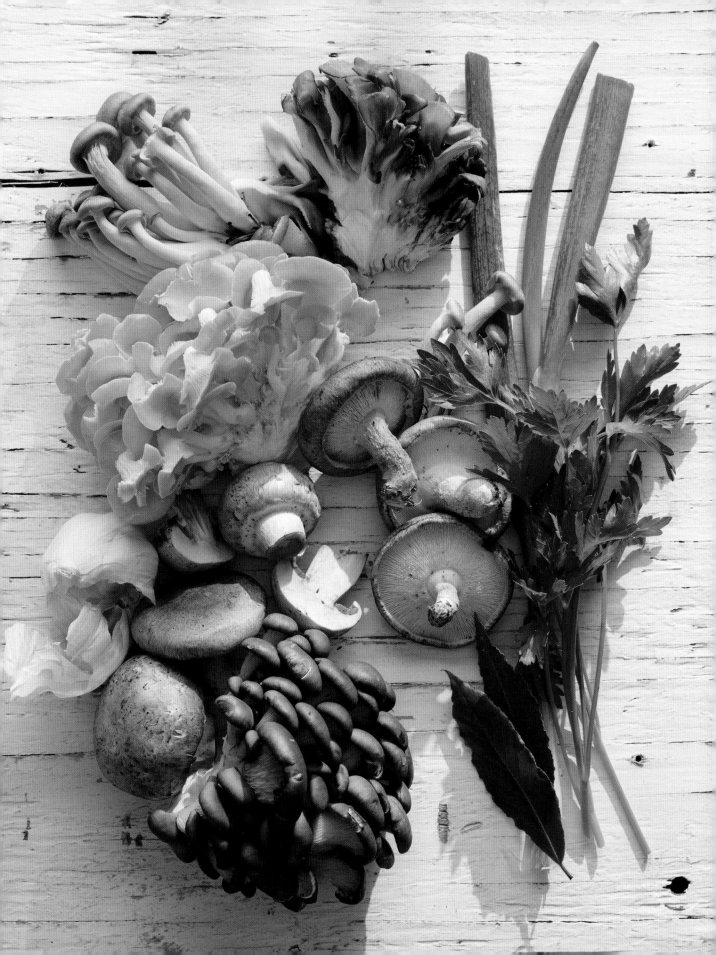

Pantry

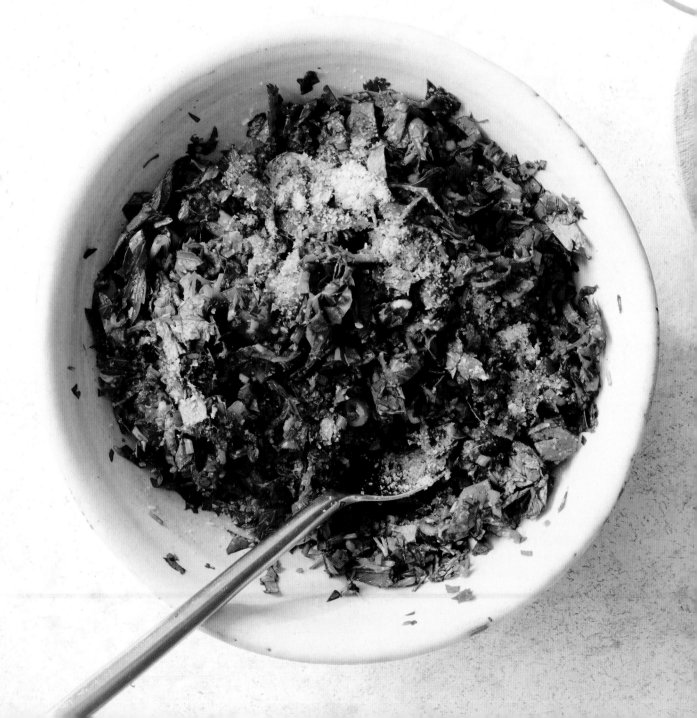

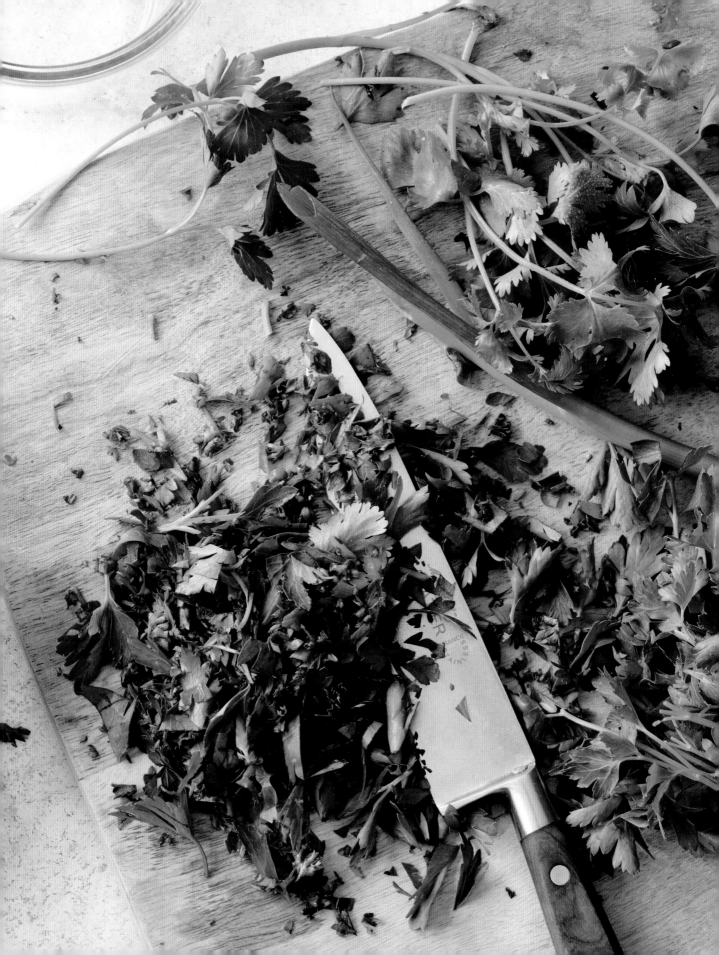

Midsummer Compote

Makes 4¼ cups

Total Time: 25 min.

6 medium black plums, pitted (1¼ lb.)

3 cups sweet cherries, pitted (1 lb.)

⅓ cup sugar

One 1-in. piece fresh ginger, peeled and thinly sliced

1¼ cups sour cherries, pitted (½ lb.)

1½ tsp. vanilla extract

Ginger, which contains melatonin, is both an anti-inflammatory food and an antioxidant. It is known to soothe nausea and reduce discomfort from menstrual cramping, osteoarthritis, and postexercise muscle pain.

Both melatonin and serotonin are found in cherries, the main ingredients of this bright summer compote. Sour cherries (also known as tart cherries) are more delicate and quicker cooking than their sweeter brethren and usually appear in markets in June and July. If you can't find them, you can use all sweet cherries (such as Bing or Rainier) instead—just be sure to dial back the sugar to 2 to 3 tablespoons. Feel free either to remove the spicy ginger pieces before serving, or nibble on them.

1. In a medium pot, stir together the plums, sweet cherries, sugar, and ginger. Set over medium heat, cover, and cook, stirring frequently, until the fruit releases its liquid, comes up to a simmer, and the plums have softened, about 10 minutes.

2. Uncover, add the sour cherries, and continue cooking, stirring occasionally, until both the sweet and sour cherries are softened, about 5 minutes more. Remove from heat, stir in the vanilla, and set aside to cool to room temperature. Transfer to an airtight container and refrigerate for up to 5 days or freeze for up to 6 months. Serve warm, chilled, or at room temperature.

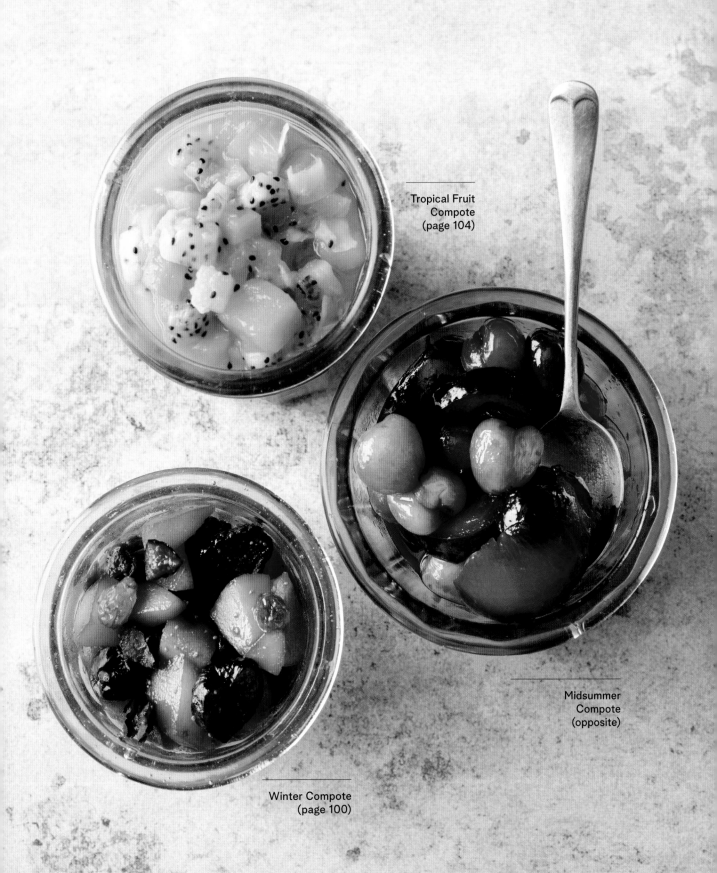

Tropical Fruit
Compote
(page 104)

Midsummer
Compote
(opposite)

Winter Compote
(page 100)

Winter Compote

Makes 2½ cups

Total Time: 35 min.

2 firm pears, peeled, cored, and coarsely chopped (⅔ lb.)

1 tart apple (such as Granny Smith or Honeycrisp), peeled, cored, and coarsely chopped (⅓ lb.)

6 dried figs, stemmed and coarsely chopped

⅓ cup dried cherries

¼ cup raisins

One 3-in. piece fresh ginger, peeled and thinly sliced

1 cinnamon stick

Two 1- by 3-in. strips fresh lemon zest

¼ cup dry red wine

3 Tbsp. honey

2 Tbsp. fresh lemon juice

Dried cherries, figs, and raisins are rich in fiber, vitamins, and minerals and cold-hardy orchard fruits like apples and pears are available year-round. Simmering these ingredients with wine, citrus, honey, and spice yields a fragrant compote that makes a cozy foundation for winter breakfast or dessert. This condiment also works nicely as an accompaniment to savory foods like cheese, roasted meats and poultry, and cold cuts.

In a medium pot, combine the pears, apple, figs, cherries, raisins, ginger, cinnamon, lemon zest, wine, honey, lemon juice, and ¼ cup of water. Bring to a boil over high heat, then lower the heat to simmer and cook, stirring frequently, until the juices thicken, the dried fruit is rehydrated, and the apples and pears are tender, 12–15 minutes. Remove from heat and cool to room temperature. Remove and discard the cinnamon stick, then transfer to an airtight container and refrigerate for up to 5 days or freeze for up to 6 months.

Tropical Fruit Compote

Makes 4 cups	Total Time: 30 min.

3 Tbsp. palm sugar

½ cup large dried coconut flakes

1½ tsp. finely grated fresh ginger

1 star anise pod

1¾ cups (¾ lb.) fresh pineapple, peeled and coarsely chopped, from one pineapple

2 medium mangoes, peeled and coarsely chopped, about 1½ cups (½ lb.)

2 kiwis, peeled and coarsely chopped, about 1 cup (⅓ lb.)

1 medium dragon fruit, peeled and coarsely chopped, about ¾ cup (⅓ lb.)

¾ tsp. vanilla extract

As this quick and sunny compote rests, the dried coconut steeps its "milk" into the juices, giving the liquid a lovely, slightly creamy texture. While the mixture may be eaten immediately after cooking, its flavor and texture are best after it has rested in the fridge for a few hours. This compote is great with breakfast and dessert, but also as a snack with yogurt, or even as a zippy accompaniment to grilled fish.

Palm sugar, derived from the sap of the coconut palm, is an unrefined sweetener with a faintly caramel flavor. Look for the soft and scoopable version, which is sold in wax-topped jars (rather than bags of rock-hard palm sugar pucks) in Asian grocery stores or online. Maple syrup or light brown sugar are good swaps, though. For the prettiest results, look for white-fleshed dragon fruit; the red-fleshed kind will taste great, too, but know that it will tint the finished mix bright pink.

In a large pot, stir together the palm sugar and ⅓ cup of water. Add the coconut, ginger, and star anise and bring to a boil over medium-high heat, stirring occasionally to dissolve the sugar. Stir in the pineapple and mango and cook until the liquid returns to a simmer, 3–4 minutes. Stir in the kiwi, bring the liquid back up to simmer again, then remove from heat and stir in the dragon fruit and vanilla extract. Cool to room temperature. Remove the star anise pod, then serve immediately or transfer to an airtight container and refrigerate for up to 5 days or freeze for up to 6 months.

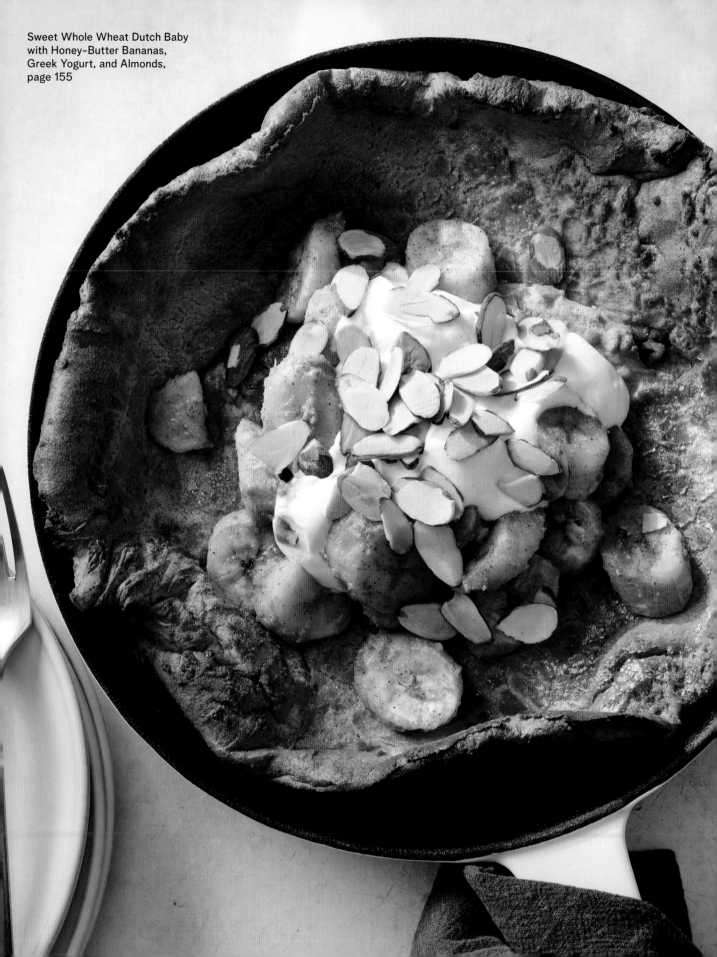

Sweet Whole Wheat Dutch Baby
with Honey-Butter Bananas,
Greek Yogurt, and Almonds,
page 155

Honey-Butter Bananas

Makes 2 cups

Total Time: 20 min.

Nonstick baking spray

4 medium bananas, sliced diagonally about ½ inch thick

⅓ cup pineapple juice

2 Tbsp. butter

2 Tbsp. honey or maple syrup

1 tsp. vanilla extract

1 tsp. ground cinnamon

¼ tsp. ground ginger

Pinch of kosher salt

We consider the banana to be one of the world's great sleep-supporting superfoods. It's a famously great source of potassium, and it is also rich in magnesium and fiber. A diet high in these three components will enhance sleep quality.

These baked bananas come together in a flash, and for such a simple recipe, they're surprisingly fragrant and delicious. Keeping a few cocktail-sized cans of pineapple juice in your pantry will allow you to whip up this sweet and nutritious condiment on the fly. Spoon over oatmeal, pancakes, a Sweet Whole Wheat Dutch Baby (page 155), yogurt, or—for an extra-special treat—vanilla or caramel ice cream. Leftovers may be stored in the fridge for a few days; rewarm gently in the microwave.

1. Position a rack in the center of the oven and preheat it to 350°F. Lightly oil a small rimmed baking sheet with nonstick baking spray. Arrange the bananas on the pan in a single layer and set aside.

2. In a small pot over medium heat, stir together the pineapple juice, butter, honey, vanilla, cinnamon, ginger, and salt. Cook gently, stirring continuously, until homogenous, then pour the mixture evenly over the bananas. Bake, rotating the pan halfway through, until the liquid is thickened and syrupy and the bananas are sticky and glazed, 15–18 minutes. Serve warm.

Sesame-Cashew Crunch

Makes 3½ cups

Total Time: 35 min.

1⅓ cups cashews,
finely chopped

⅔ cup sesame seeds

¼ cup oat bran

½ cup honey

1 Tbsp. olive or vegetable oil

1 tsp. sesame oil

½ tsp. flaky sea salt

Use this shaggy, tryptophan-rich brittle as a snack or crunchy topping for savory dishes like salads or roasted root vegetables, breakfast foods like hot cereal and smoothie bowls, or even desserts like ice cream, baked fruit, or pudding—essentially, anywhere you would add a sprinkling of nuts.

1. Preheat the oven to 350°F. Line a large rimmed baking sheet with parchment or foil and set aside.

2. In a large bowl, stir together the cashews, sesame seeds, and oat bran. Set aside.

3. In a large pot over medium heat, stir together the honey and oils and cook, swirling occasionally, until the liquid is hot and beginning to simmer. Remove from heat, then pour over the cashew mixture and stir to combine.

4. Turn the cashew mixture out onto the prepared baking sheet and spread into an even layer. Sprinkle with salt, then bake, using a fork to occasionally stir and fluff, until the nuts and seeds turn a deep golden brown, 15–20 minutes. (The mixture will still seem sticky and wet, but it will crisp up as it cools.) Set aside to cool to room temperature, then use immediately or transfer to an airtight jar and store at room temperature for up to 1 month.

Beet Hummus

Makes 2⅓ cups

Total Time: 45 min.

3 medium beets
(½ lb.), scrubbed

6 whole peeled garlic cloves

One 15.5-oz. can chickpeas,
rinsed and drained

¼ cup tahini

2 Tbsp. fresh lemon juice

1 Tbsp. extra-virgin olive
oil, plus more as needed

Kosher salt

White and black sesame
seeds, for garnish

Beets are particularly rich in
naturally occurring nitrate
(not to be confused with
nitrites, the preservatives
used in processed meats).
Our body converts nitrate to
nitric oxide, which relaxes
our blood vessels, improving
blood flow and reducing blood
pressure. In a 2020 study of
folks suffering from chronic
obstructive pulmonary disease
(COPD), a glass of beet juice
in the evening normalized sleep
architecture (transitions from
one sleep stage to the next) in
these patients.

Homemade hummus is much less expensive than store-bought versions, and you can also easily customize the simple dip with additional sleep-supporting ingredients. Blitzing in a few colorful cooked beets adds magnesium and folate, and a generous drizzle of tahini provides richness, tryptophan, and gamma-aminobutyric acid (GABA), a known stress-reducer—and of course less stress will help you fall asleep faster. Tahini is a popular, Middle Eastern-style sesame paste, but Chinese- and Japanese-style sesame pastes may be substituted here as well. Try to find whole seed versions; these styles tend to be richer in calcium, fiber, and iron than sesame pastes made from hulled seeds. If garlic is a heartburn trigger for you, feel free to dial back the quantity used, or omit it entirely.

1. In a small pot, combine the beets, garlic, and enough cold water to cover by 1 inch. Bring to a boil over medium-high heat and cook, stirring occasionally, until the beets are tender when poked with a paring knife, 30–40 minutes. Using a slotted spoon, transfer the garlic cloves to the bowl of a food processor. Transfer the beets to a heatproof bowl and set aside, reserving the cooking liquid.

2. When the beets are cool enough to handle, use a few layers of paper towels to remove and discard the skins. Add the beets to the food processor, along with the chickpeas, tahini, lemon juice, and olive oil. Process until smooth, thinning with up to ¼ cup of the reserved beet-cooking liquid if needed. Season to taste with kosher salt, then transfer the hummus to an airtight container and chill until ready to eat, at least 2 hours. Leftovers will keep for up to 4 days. To serve, drizzle with a bit more olive oil and sprinkle with sesame seeds.

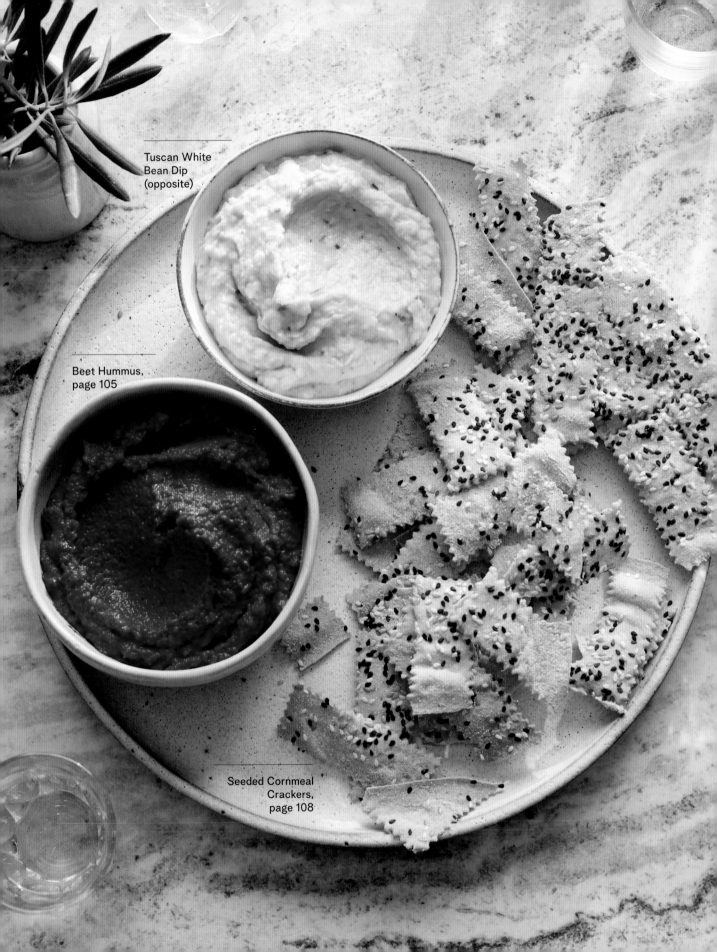

Tuscan White
Bean Dip
(opposite)

Beet Hummus,
page 105

Seeded Cornmeal
Crackers,
page 108

Tuscan White Bean Dip

Makes 2½ cups

Total Time: 15 min.

Two 15.5-oz. cans cannellini beans, rinsed and drained

2 garlic cloves, coarsely chopped

1 Tbsp. finely chopped fresh rosemary (or substitute 1 tsp. dried rosemary)

1 tsp. finely grated lemon zest

2 Tbsp. fresh lemon juice

2 Tbsp. extra-virgin olive oil

Kosher salt and freshly ground black pepper

White beans are another sleep-supporting superfood: The humble legume is a great source of dietary tryptophan and fiber as well as three of the four essential nutrients that support our body's production of serotonin and melatonin—folate, magnesium, and zinc.

This silky and aromatic bean dip comes together quickly using just a handful of pantry ingredients. Spread it over toast and top with crispy baked kale or serve with crudités for a flavorful and low-fuss vegan appetizer. Or portion it into plastic containers for a convenient, on-the-go protein source. Extra-virgin olive oil is an anti-inflammatory food that's rich in sleep-healthy monounsaturated fatty acids; if you have a robustly flavored, high-quality bottle, this is the place to use it.

In the bowl of a food processor, combine the beans, ¼ cup of water, garlic, rosemary, and lemon zest. Process until finely chopped, then, with the motor running, drizzle in the lemon juice followed by olive oil. (Stop processing to scrape down the sides and bottom of the bowl a few times.) Season to taste with kosher salt and freshly ground black pepper and continue processing until very smooth. If the purée seems dry, add additional water a tablespoon at a time until you reach a silky, whipped consistency. Serve immediately or transfer to an airtight container and refrigerate for up to 4 days.

Seeded Cornmeal Crackers

Makes about 60 crackers

Total Time: 1 hr., plus 4 hr. to rest the dough

1 tsp. instant yeast

1 tsp. honey

1 cup corn flour (115 g), plus more for dusting

¾ cup all-purpose flour (105 g)

¼ cup whole wheat flour (35 g)

2 Tbsp. extra-virgin olive oil, plus more for greasing

1 tsp. fine sea salt

1 Tbsp. flaxseeds

1 Tbsp. sesame seeds

1 Tbsp. nigella seeds (or substitute black sesame seeds)

Flaky sea salt

Nigella—also known as *Nigella sativa*, or black seed—has long been used as a culinary and medicinal ingredient in Mediterranean and Asian cultures. It has a savory and faintly smoky flavor; if you can't find it (or don't like it!), feel free to substitute black sesame seeds instead.

The trick to these wonderfully crisp and delicate crackers is to roll them paper-thin and bake them very gently—they should take on almost no color at all in the oven. Corn flour (*not* to be confused with cornstarch) is a whole grain flour, which lends this cracker dough layers of flavor and texture. Bob's Red Mill sells a reliable version, but if you can't find it, you can just blitz ordinary cornmeal in a blender or food processor until it is powdery.

1. In the bowl of a stand mixer fitted with a dough hook, stir together ¾ cup of water and the yeast and honey. Add the three flours, olive oil, and fine sea salt, then mix on low speed until a dough forms, 1–2 minutes. Increase the speed to medium and continue mixing until the dough is smooth and shiny, 5–6 minutes (it will still be a bit sticky). If you don't have a mixer, this can be done by hand: In the same order, add the ingredients to a large bowl. Using a fork or dough whisk, mix until a shaggy dough forms, then, using lightly oiled hands, knead the dough in the bowl until it is smooth and shiny, about 10 minutes.

2. If you are using a mixer, remove the hook and remove the bowl from the base. Cover the bowl tightly with plastic wrap and refrigerate for at least 4 hours and up to a day. (If making the dough in advance, it may also be transferred to a zip-top freezer bag, then stored, frozen, for up to a month.)

3. Position a rack in the center of the oven and preheat it to 300°F. In a small bowl, stir together the flax, sesame, and nigella seeds; season lightly with flaky sea salt.

4. Remove the dough from the fridge and divide it into thirds. Generously dust a large sheet of parchment paper with corn flour, then place one third of the dough atop it; generously dust the surface of the dough with more corn flour, then, using a rolling pin, roll the dough out to a very thin layer, adding more corn flour as needed to prevent sticking as you go. Using a pastry brush, brush the surface of the dough lightly with cold water, then sprinkle evenly with a third of the seed mixture. Roll once or twice lightly to press the seeds into the dough, then prick the dough all over with a fork. Using a large chef's knife, a fluted pastry wheel, or a pizza cutter, score the sheet into approximately 1- by 3-inch rectangles (don't bother pulling the individual crackers apart).

5. Use the parchment paper to slide the sheet of dough onto a large rimmed baking sheet. Bake, rotating the pan once halfway through cooking, until crisp and very lightly golden, 20–25 minutes.

6. Repeat with the remaining remaining cracker dough and seed mixture. Cool the crackers to room temperature, then break apart and serve immediately or transfer to an airtight container and store in a cool, dry place for up to 7 days.

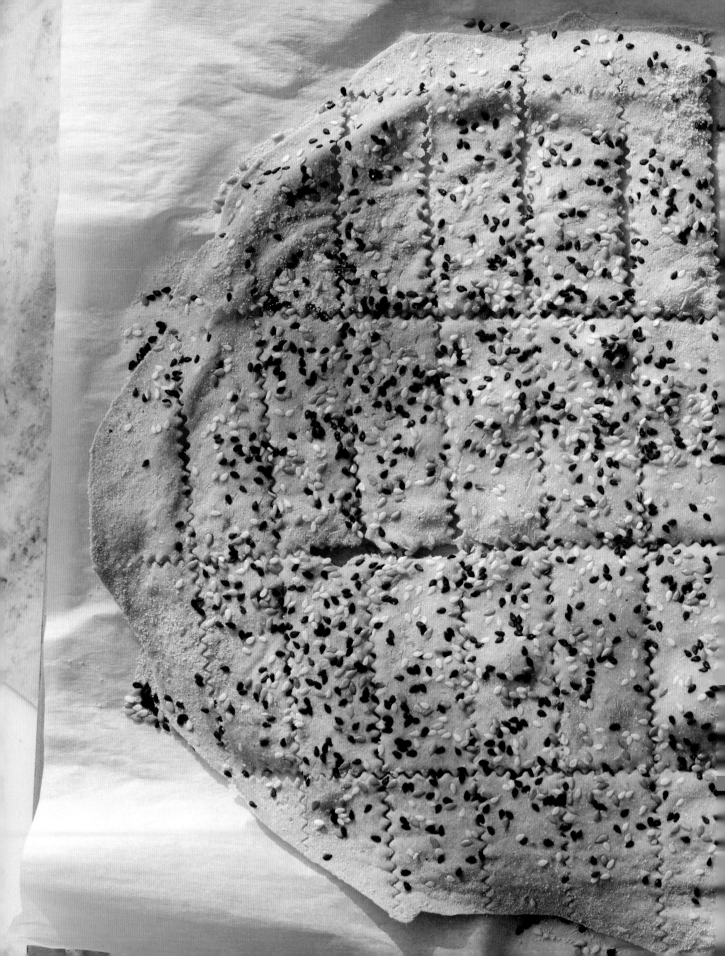

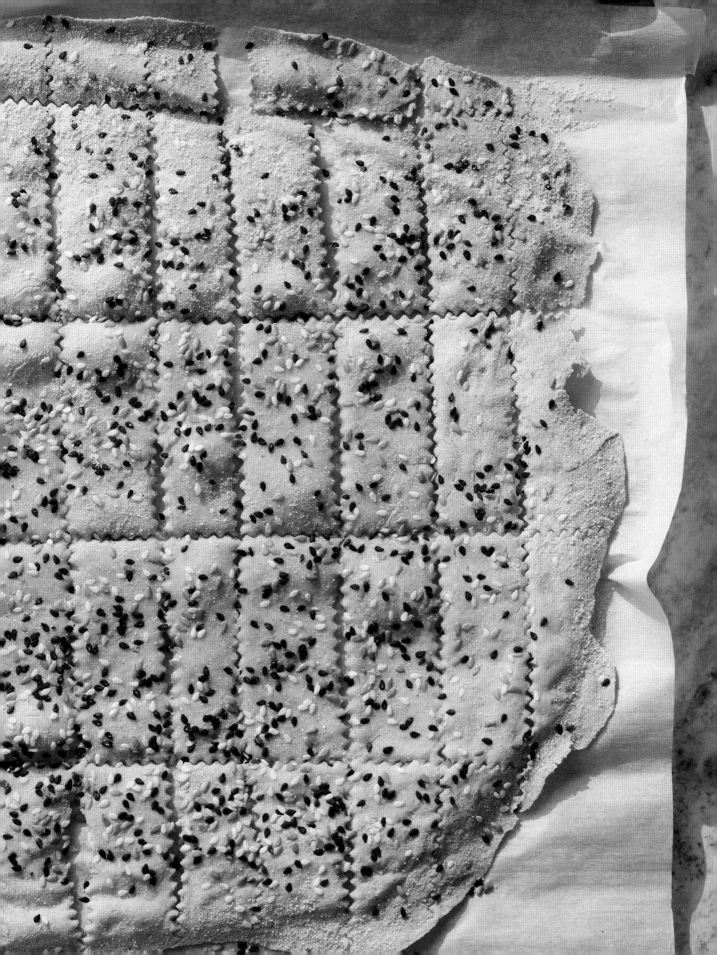

Sesame-Sunflower Oat Bread

Makes one 9-in. loaf

Total Time: 1 hr. 30 min., plus 2 hr. fermentation

1 cup plus 1½ tsp. buttermilk, divided

1 Tbsp. honey

2¼ tsp. instant yeast

⅓ cup rolled (old-fashioned) oats (35 g)

2 Tbsp. oat bran

3 Tbsp. olive oil, plus more for greasing

2¼ cups all-purpose flour (295 g), plus more for kneading

1 cup whole wheat flour (120 g)

1¼ tsp. fine sea salt

2 Tbsp. sunflower seeds

3 Tbsp sesame seeds, divided

If the thought of baking your own bread sounds stressful and exhausting, feel free to turn the page. There are plenty of bakeries out there making delicious, healthy loaves loaded with sleep-supporting whole grains and seeds. However, if you enjoy baking like we do, you might find hand-mixing this simple sandwich loaf to be a relaxing weekend activity.

We intentionally included plenty of tryptophan-rich ingredients in this recipe. Feel free to swap out the whole wheat flour for spelt or other heirloom flours if you like, but don't mess with the white bread flour, which is high in protein and the key to a soft and fluffy loaf. Be sure to use dried yeast labeled either *instant* or *rapid rise*. Unlike dry active yeast, these more finely powdered types do not need to be bloomed in warm water and can go right into the dough. Remember that ambient temperature, humidity, and differences in water and flour all have an impact on yeast development; the fermentation and rising times listed are approximations and we suggest paying attention to visual and tactile cues as you go. On a warm summer day, this recipe may move much more quickly than in the dead of winter.

This recipe riffs on porridge bread, in which the dough includes a portion of cooked or soaked cereal grains. The technique allows you to sneak more hydration into the loaf, resulting in a bread that stays soft and fresh longer than breads made using a straight mix. However, know that, unlike packaged loaves, this one doesn't contain preservatives that fend off mold. If storing it for longer than 3 days, wrap it tightly in plastic wrap and freeze.

1. In a large bowl, stir together 1 cup of buttermilk, ¼ cup of cool water, and the honey and yeast. Stir in the oats and oat bran and set aside until the oats are hydrated, about 15 minutes.

—continued—

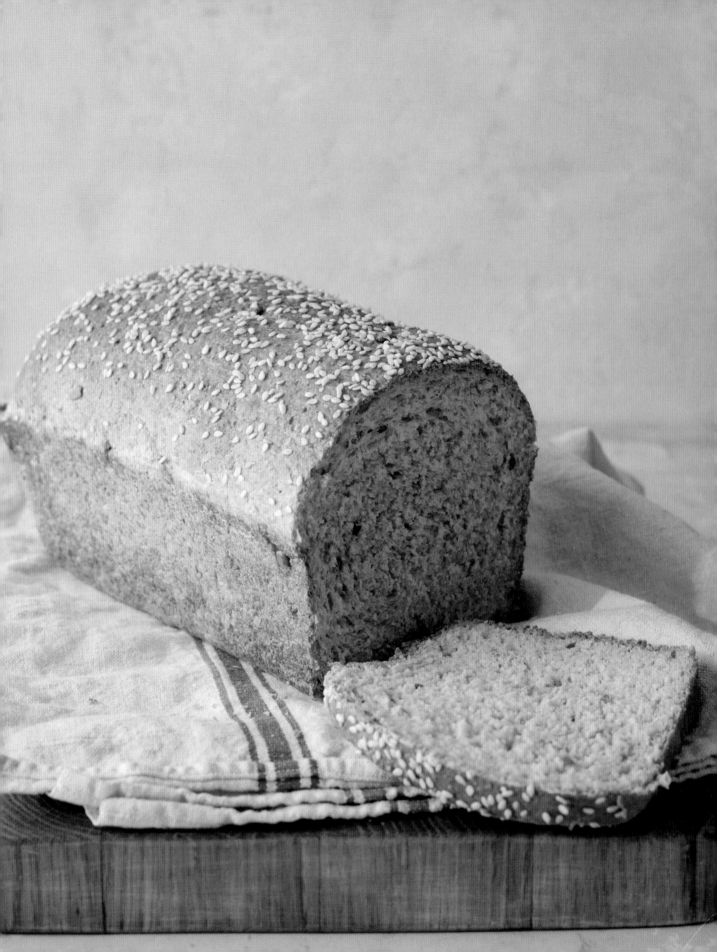

2. Add the olive oil, flours, and salt and, using a wooden spoon or silicone spatula, stir until a shaggy dough begins to form. Lightly flour a clean work surface, turn the dough out onto it, then knead until smooth, about 7 minutes (the dough should clean your work surface and not stick). Lightly oil a medium bowl, place the dough in it, and cover with a lid or plastic wrap. Set aside in a warm place until the dough is very soft and is beginning to feel airy (it will not yet be doubled in size), 20–25 minutes.

3. Lightly flour your work surface again, turn the dough out onto it, and stretch and lightly press it down to make an even ½-inch-thick circle. Sprinkle the dough evenly with the sunflower seeds and 2 tablespoons of sesame seeds, then give the dough a few quick kneads to distribute the seeds. Shape it into a loose ball and return the dough to the greased bowl, cover, and set aside until the dough is once again soft and airy, 30–35 minutes more.

4. Lightly grease a 9- by 5-inch loaf pan. Turn the dough out onto the work surface and press it down to an even disk. Fold the left and right sides in over each other, then pull and stretch the top edge over and down 3 times to make an approximately 8-inch-long loaf shape. Place the loaf, seam-side down, in the prepared loaf pan, cover loosely with plastic wrap, and set aside in a warm place until puffed and just barely doubled in size, 60–70 minutes.

5. Meanwhile, position a rack in the bottom third of the oven and preheat it to 375°F. In a small bowl, whisk the remaining 1½ teaspoons of buttermilk with 1½ teaspoons of cool water.

6. When the loaf has risen, uncover and, using a pastry brush, coat the surface evenly with the buttermilk-water mixture. Sprinkle liberally with the remaining tablespoon of sesame seeds, then transfer to the oven. Immediately lower the temperature to 350°F and bake until evenly golden brown, 40–45 minutes. Cool for 10 minutes in the pan, then pop the loaf out, place on a wire rack, and finish cooling to room temperature before slicing.

Creamy Sesame-Ginger Vinaigrette

Makes ¾ cup

Total Time: 5 min.

3 Tbsp. extra-virgin olive oil

1 Tbsp. sesame oil

2 Tbsp. low-sodium soy sauce

2 Tbsp. rice vinegar

1 Tbsp. honey

One 2-in. piece fresh ginger, finely chopped

1 Tbsp. tahini

2 tsp. sesame seeds

You may notice that we use a lot of tahini in this book. That's because sesame is a sleep-supporting superfood rich in tryptophan, gamma-aminobutyric acid (GABA), fiber, zinc, and other essential nutrients. Sesame tahini is made from sesame seeds that have been ground to a smooth paste; it can be used as a base for rich and creamy sauces. Like all-natural nut butters, tahini tends to separate as it sits, so give it a good stir with a spoon or chopstick before using.

This sweet-and-savory dressing is low in saturated fat and rich in heart-healthy (and sleep-healthy) monounsaturated and polyunsaturated fats. We love it added to a simple green salad, cold noodles, roasted chicken, or grilled or broiled fish.

In a blender or small food processor, combine the olive oil, sesame oil, soy sauce, vinegar, honey, ginger, tahini, and 2 tablespoons of water and process until smooth. (Alternatively, combine the ingredients in a small bowl and beat with a hand blender, eggbeater, or whisk until smooth.) Transfer to a bowl or jar, stir in the sesame seeds, and use immediately or cover and refrigerate for up to 2 weeks.

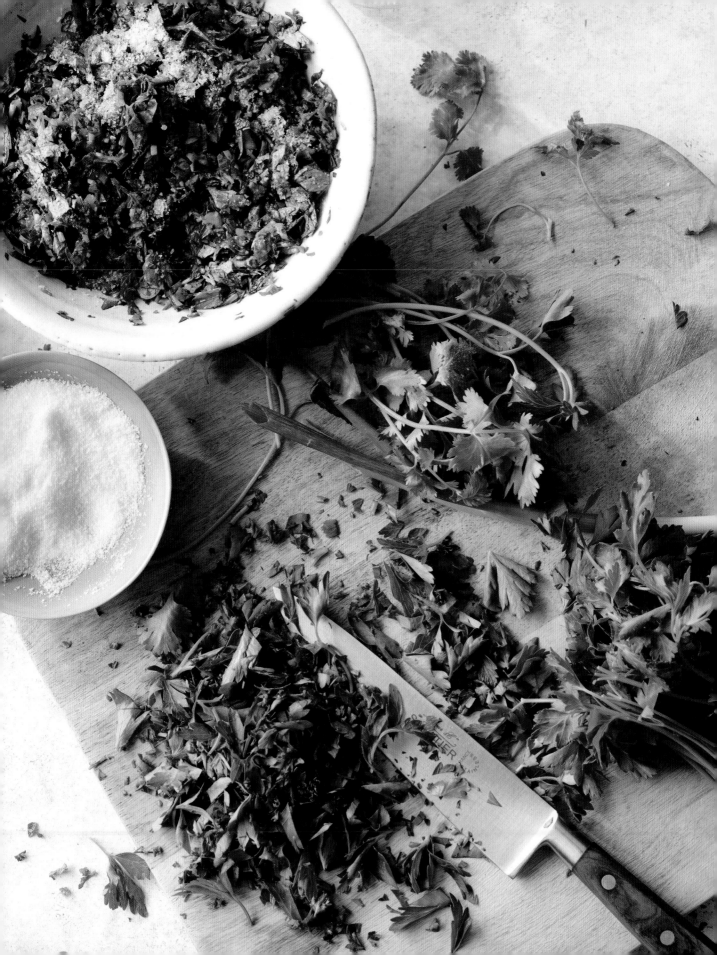

Herbes Salées

Makes 2 cups | Total Time: 5 min.

2½ cups coarsely chopped fresh parsley

1 cup coarsely chopped fresh cilantro

¾ cup thinly sliced scallions (both white and green parts) (about 7 scallions)

¼ cup kosher salt

Fresh herbs are a marvelous and inexpensive way to elevate even the simplest foods with vibrance and flavor. But it can be difficult to make it through bunches of potent herbs before they turn swampy in the fridge. Enter: herbes salées. Simply "salted herbs," this traditional Quebecois seasoning uses a basic preservation technique—salt!—to save that mountain of fresh herbs for weeks. This basic formula calls for a mix of parsley, cilantro, and scallions, but you can swap in chives, chervil, dill, or any other soft-stemmed herbs that you like. Use a teaspoon or two of this mixture anywhere you would otherwise add a tablespoon of chopped fresh herbs; just remember to go easy on the salt and always adjust the seasoning to taste.

In a large bowl, toss together the parsley, cilantro, scallions, and salt. Use immediately or pack into jars, cover tightly, and refrigerate for up to 3 months. Stir by the spoonful into soups, stews, salad dressings, and sauces.

Pickled Mushrooms

Makes about 3 cups | Total Time: 15 min., plus 24 hr. to pickle

1⅓ lb. assorted fresh
mushrooms, brushed
clean, ends trimmed

1 Tbsp. kosher salt, plus
more for boiling (divided)

1 medium scallion, trimmed,
halved lengthwise

2 sprigs fresh parsley

2 bay leaves

1 medium garlic clove,
halved and lightly crushed

¼ tsp. crushed red chile
flakes (optional)

¼ tsp. dried thyme

1¼ cups sherry vinegar

1 Tbsp. honey or maple syrup

This zippy and umami-rich condiment is especially good with a mix of mushrooms, but even the ordinary white button variety is delicious. If you are using shiitakes, be sure to remove their stems as they are too tough to eat. (Shiitake stems and other mushroom trimmings may be frozen or dried and saved for adding flavor to stocks and broths.)

Sherry vinegar is less dark and syrupy than balsamic, with a balanced sweetness and gentle acidity. If you can't find it, feel free to substitute apple cider vinegar or equal parts red wine vinegar and white wine vinegar. Save the leftover mushroom-cooking liquid for adding to soups, stews, and risotto.

1. Cut the mushrooms into bite-sized pieces: Button mushrooms and cremini can be halved or quartered, while more delicate wild mushrooms like hen-of-the-woods and oyster mushrooms can be torn into pieces. Set aside.

2. Bring a large pot of lightly salted water to a boil, then boil the mushrooms until tender, 5–7 minutes. Drain and pack the mushrooms into two 16-ounce heatproof jars along with the scallion, parsley, bay leaves, garlic, chile flakes, if using, and thyme.

3. In a small pot over medium heat, bring the vinegar, honey, 1 tablespoon of salt, and ½ cup of water to a boil. Pour the brine over the mushrooms to submerge, then screw on the lids, cool to room temperature, and refrigerate for at least 24 hours before using. The mushrooms will keep well in the fridge for at least a month.

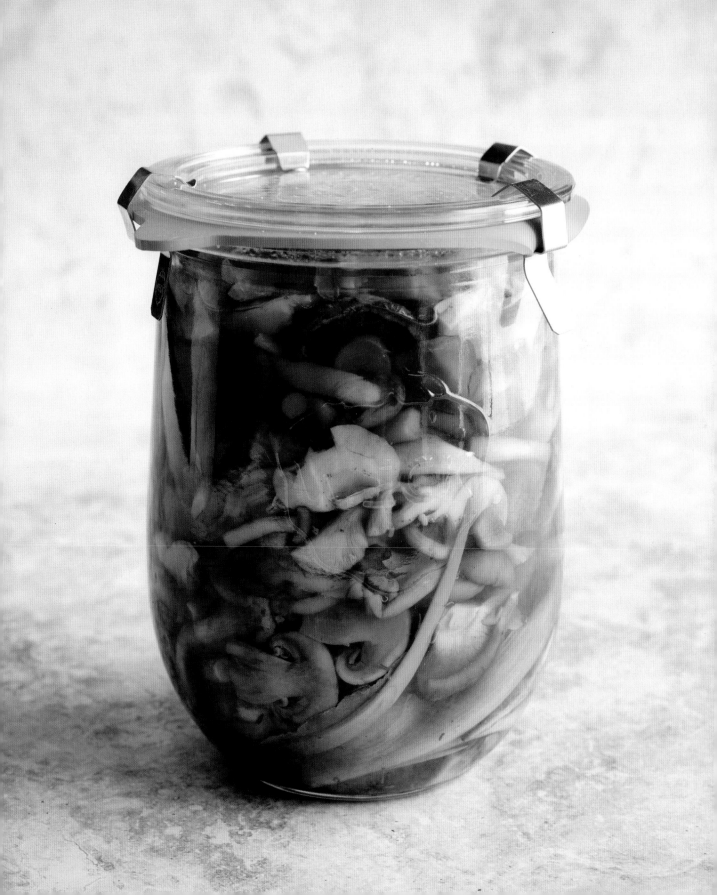

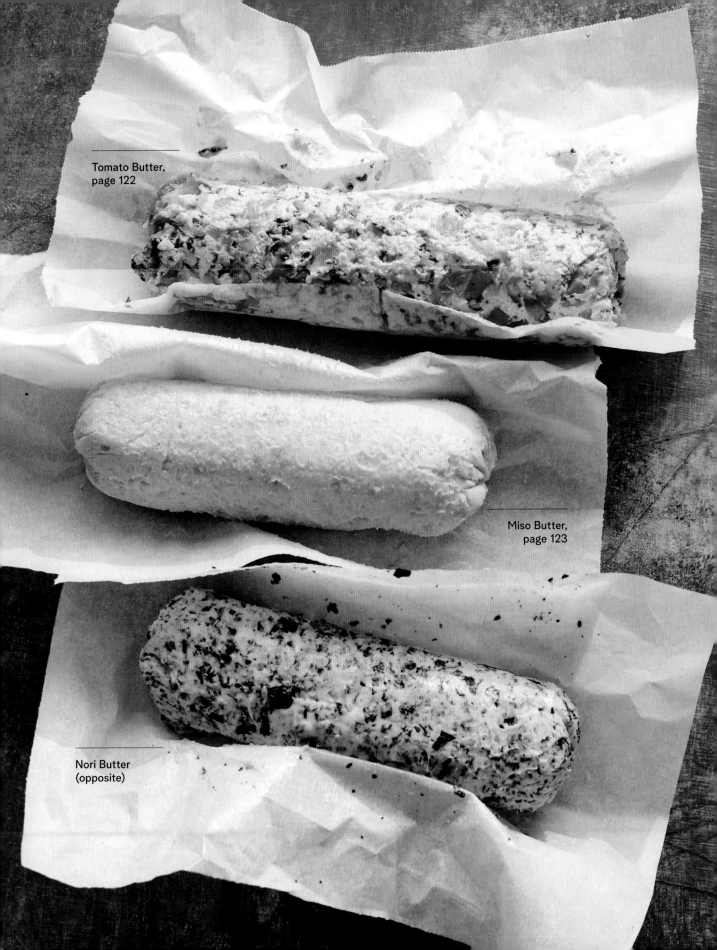

Tomato Butter,
page 122

Miso Butter,
page 123

Nori Butter
(opposite)

Three Compound Butters

We know that healthy fat is important for healthy brain function and healthy sleep—but a diet high in saturated fat is associated with less overall deep sleep than one higher in monounsaturated and polyunsaturated fats.

But butter tastes really good, right? Compound butter is a nice way to sneak the taste of butter into your diet while diluting its saturated fat content with some flavorful (and sleep-supporting!) ingredients. Still, use these butters sparingly, as a finishing touch. They all keep well in the freezer for several months.

Nori Butter

Makes 1⅓ cups

Total Time: 10 min.

1 cup (2 sticks) softened unsalted butter

Three 8- by 7½-inch sheets roasted nori, torn into small pieces

2 tsp. fresh lemon juice

2 tsp. sesame oil

½ tsp. kosher salt

2 Tbsp. sesame seeds

This umami-rich seaweed butter is wonderful melted over fish, shellfish, or roasted vegetables. Like all leafy greens, seaweeds are packed with fiber and essential nutrients. Since nori is the most widely available seaweed in conventional American grocery stores, we went with it for this recipe. (You may recognize the thin, pressed sheets from sushi restaurants, where nori is used to wrap maki.) However, sustainably raised domestic seaweed production is on the rise, so if you have access to other types, by all means feel free to swap in another dried or fresh variety. We're especially fond of dulse for its pretty purple hue and bacony flavor; thicker, tougher seaweeds like kelp should be rehydrated in water and finely chopped before using.

In a food processor, combine the butter, nori, lemon juice, sesame oil, and salt, then process, scraping down the sides and bottom of the bowl as needed, until the butter is very smooth and the ingredients are incorporated. Add the sesame seeds and pulse to incorporate, then transfer the butter to a jar or form into logs and wrap tightly in plastic wrap. Refrigerate until firm and use within 2 weeks or freeze for up to 6 months.

Tomato Butter

Makes 2 cups	Total Time: 40 min.

2 medium beefsteak tomatoes (about 1 lb.), coarsely chopped

1 Tbsp. extra-virgin olive oil

¾ tsp. kosher salt

½ tsp. dried oregano

¼ tsp. garlic powder

Pinch of crushed red chile flakes (optional)

Freshly ground black pepper

½ cup loosely packed fresh basil leaves

1 cup (2 sticks) softened unsalted butter

Tomatoes—particularly the big and meaty beefsteak variety—contain both melatonin and serotonin, so we try to fit this flavorful sleep-supporting ingredient into our diet wherever we can. Freezing a batch of this compound butter is a great way to preserve the goodness of your peak-season garden or farmers' market haul through the winter.

1. Position a rack in the center of the oven and preheat it to 425°F.

2. Line a large rimmed baking sheet with parchment or foil. Add the tomatoes, drizzle with olive oil, then sprinkle with the salt, oregano, garlic powder, chile flakes, if using, and black pepper. Toss to coat, then roast until the tomatoes are beginning to caramelize slightly and their juices are concentrated and bubbling, 20–25 minutes. Set aside to cool completely to room temperature.

3. Scrape the tomatoes and any accumulated juices into the bowl of a food processor. Add the basil and pulse just until finely chopped, but not completely puréed. Add the butter, a few tablespoons at a time, scraping down the bowl and blade occasionally, until completely combined. Transfer to a jar or form into logs and wrap tightly in plastic wrap. Refrigerate until firm and use within a week or freeze for up to 6 months.

Miso Butter

Makes 1½ cups	Total Time: 10 min.

1 cup (2 sticks) softened unsalted butter

⅓ cup miso

Miso is a salted and fermented soybean paste traditionally used as a soup base or seasoning in Japan. It sometimes also contains grains like rice or barley. We used a reduced-sodium brown rice miso for this recipe, but you may swap in any type.

Place the butter and miso in the bowl of a food processor and process to combine, scraping down the sides and bottom of the bowl as needed, until the butter is very smooth and the miso is fully incorporated. Transfer to a jar or form into logs and wrap tightly in plastic wrap. Refrigerate until firm and use within 2 weeks or freeze for up to 6 months.

Simple Baked Sweet Potato with Miso Butter

Position a rack in the center of the oven and preheat it to 450°F. Line a baking sheet with parchment or foil. Prick a **medium sweet potato** all over with a fork, then place it on the baking sheet and bake until tender when poked in the center with a thin paring knife, 40–50 minutes. Remove from the oven, cool slightly, then split the potato lengthwise on one side. Lightly mash the flesh with a fork, top with **a tablespoon of Miso Butter**, **a tablespoon of thinly sliced scallions**, and **a big pinch of sesame seeds**. Serve hot.

Two Salsas

Alliums and peppers are considered anti-inflammatory foods, while tomatoes contain both serotonin and melatonin. These delicious and nutrient-rich ingredients feature prominently in our sleep-healthy plan. However, we also recognize that these can be common heartburn triggers for some. If you find these ingredients are disrupting your sleep, avoid them after noon. For more on this, see "Indigestion and Acid Reflux" (page 56).

Salsa Roja

Makes 3 cups | Total Time: 15 min.

2 large beefsteak tomatoes (about 1 lb.), halved

½ medium white onion, peeled and halved

2 medium dried guajillo or ancho chiles, stemmed, seeded, and soaked in hot water until pliable

¼ cup coarsely chopped fresh cilantro leaves and stems

2 tsp. dried oregano

1 tsp. ground coriander

1 tsp. ground cumin

1 Tbsp. fresh lime juice

Kosher salt

This rich and roasted condiment can be customized to any heat level you like. If you prefer a milder flavor, stick with guajillo chiles and remove all of the seeds. For a bit more heat, use ancho chiles instead. If you like your salsa extra hot, leave in some or all of the chile seeds.

Heat a large, well-seasoned or lightly oiled cast-iron skillet, griddle, or grill pan over medium-high heat, then arrange the tomatoes and onion on it, cut-side down. Cook, without moving, until charred, 4–7 minutes, then turn and continue cooking until the tomato skins are lightly charred as well, 2–4 minutes more. Transfer the tomatoes and onion to a blender. Add the chiles, cilantro, oregano, coriander, cumin, and lime juice. Pulse to blend to a chunky sauce, then season to taste with salt. Transfer to a bowl, cool to room temperature, and use immediately or pack into an airtight jar and refrigerate for up to 1 week.

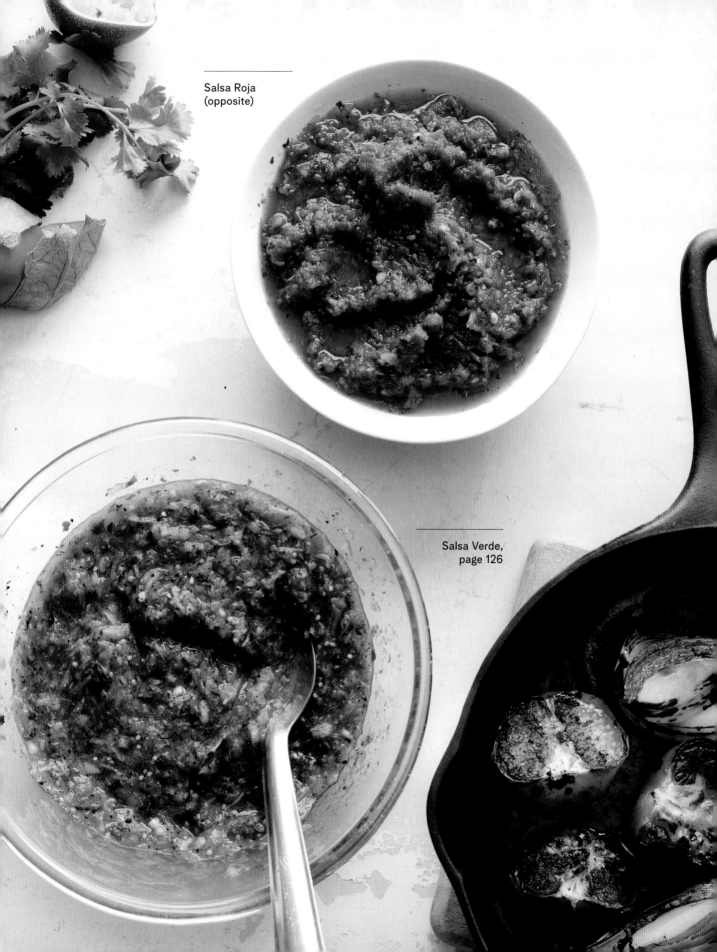

Salsa Roja
(opposite)

Salsa Verde,
page 126

Salsa Verde

Makes 2½ cups	Total Time: 30 min.

½ medium white onion, peeled and halved

2 serrano chiles

¾ lb. tomatillos, husks removed, halved

½ cup coarsely chopped fresh cilantro

2 medium scallions, trimmed and coarsely chopped

1 tsp. ground coriander

1 tsp. ground cumin

1 Tbsp. fresh lime juice

Kosher salt

This tart green tomatillo sauce shines alongside poultry, beef, or pork. Seek out firm-fleshed and unblemished tomatillos, which are typically sold still in their papery husks.

1. Heat a large, well-seasoned or lightly oiled cast-iron skillet, griddle, or grill pan over medium-high heat. Add the onion and chiles and cook, turning occasionally, until charred all over, 5–7 minutes. As the vegetables are finished (the onion will take longer than the chiles), transfer to a cutting board and set aside until cool enough to handle.

2. Coarsely chop the onion. Stem the chiles and remove and discard their seeds. (If you prefer a spicier salsa, you may leave some or all of the seeds in.) Transfer the vegetables to a blender.

3. Return the skillet to medium-high heat and add the tomatillos, cut side down. Cook, without moving, until lightly charred, 3–4 minutes, then turn and continue cooking until the skins are lightly charred as well, 3–4 minutes more. Transfer to the blender, then add the cilantro, scallions, coriander, cumin, and lime juice. Pulse to blend to a chunky sauce, then season to taste with salt. Transfer to a bowl, cool to room temperature, and use immediately or pack into an airtight jar and refrigerate for up to 1 week.

Garlicky Fish Sauce Dressing

Makes ⅔ cup

Total Time: 15 min.

½ cup finely chopped garlic

½ cup extra-virgin olive oil

2 Tbsp. fish sauce

1 Tbsp. sesame oil

Freshly ground black pepper

Fish sauce is used throughout East and Southeast Asia and bottled versions vary in flavor and quality. We especially like the Vietnamese brand Red Boat. This punchy recipe is adapted from the Red Boat cookbook, and we find that it is particularly tasty on sleep-healthy cruciferous vegetables, like broccoli and Brussels sprouts, and dark leafy greens. Keep a batch in the fridge, and whenever you need to get something green on the table quickly, just sauté (or even microwave) your veg lightly until wilted and tender, then toss with a splash of this savory condiment.

In a small pot over low heat, combine the garlic and olive oil and cook, swirling occasionally, until the garlic is fragrant and evenly golden, 12–14 minutes. Remove from heat, stir in the fish sauce and sesame oil, and season generously with black pepper. Use immediately or transfer to an airtight container and refrigerate for up to 2 weeks or freeze for up to 3 months. Stir well before using.

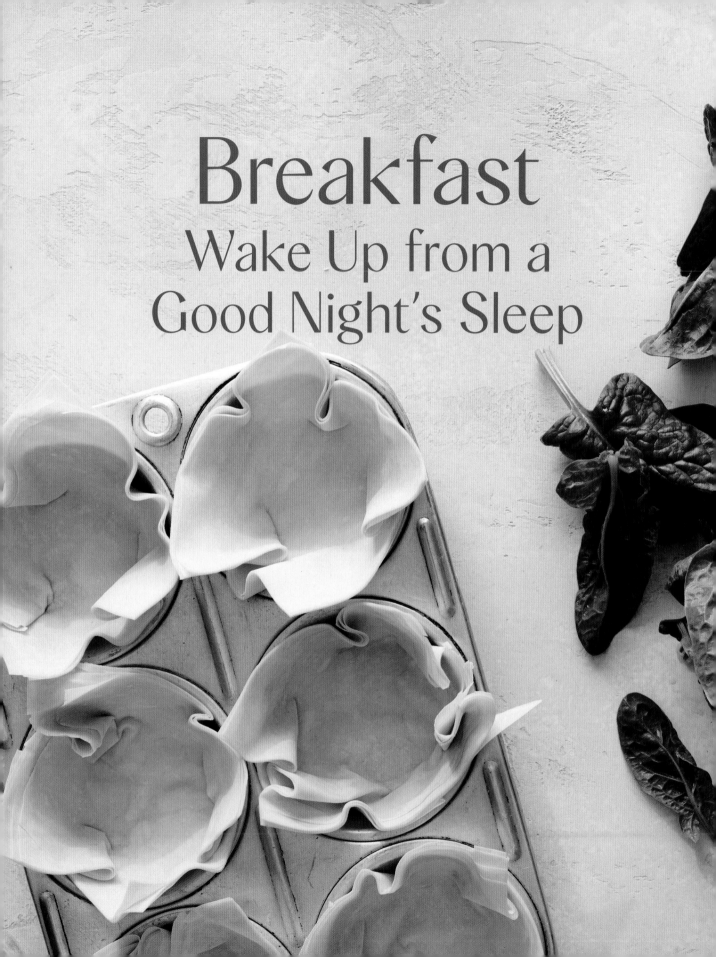

Breakfast
Wake Up from a Good Night's Sleep

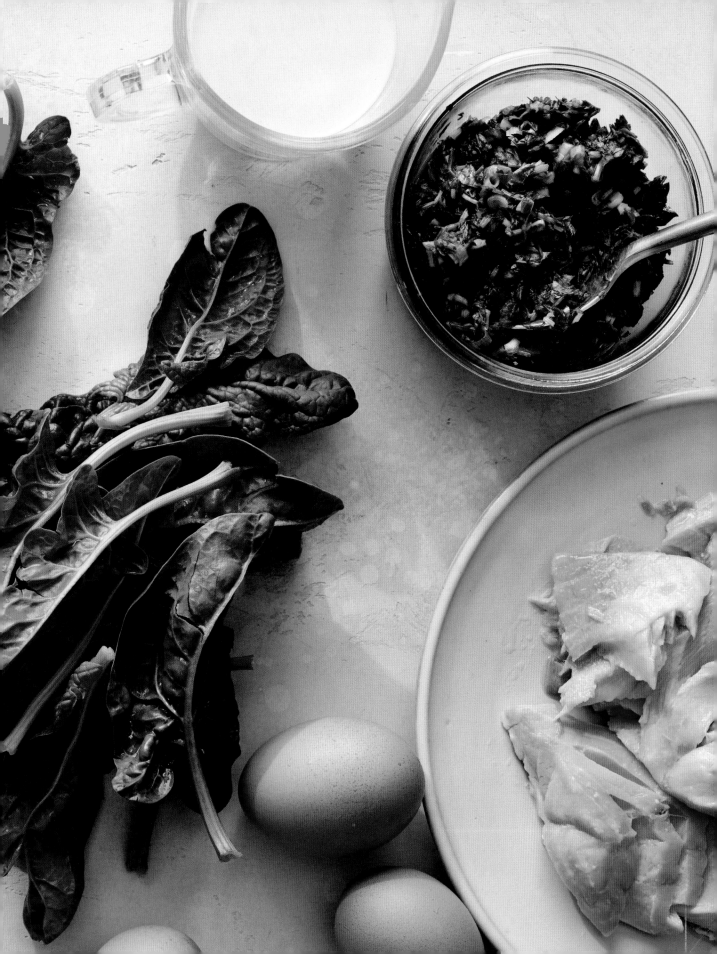

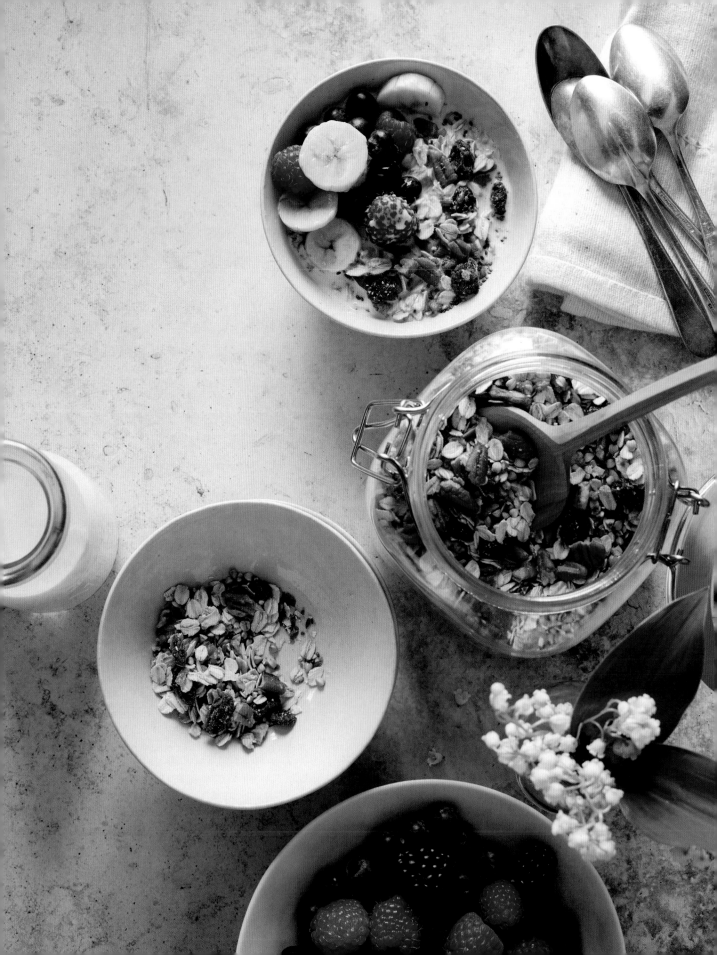

Maple-Pecan Muesli

Makes 5½ cups | Total Time: 5 min.

3 cups rolled
(old-fashioned) oats

1 cup buckwheat flakes
(such as Bob's Red Mill
Buckwheat Hot Cereal)

1 cup chopped pecans

1 cup raisins

⅓ cup maple sugar or
dark brown sugar

¼ cup chia seeds

¼ cup flaxseed

1 tsp. ground cinnamon

½ tsp. kosher salt

Mix up a batch of this Swiss-style pantry staple, which can be enjoyed as an on-the-go snack, sprinkled over a 6-ounce container of yogurt, or as the base for an overnight breakfast: Simply stir together ½ cup muesli, ½ cup dairy or plant-based milk, and ½ cup water; refrigerate for 8–24 hours; then eat cold or zap in the microwave for 45 seconds to warm. Top with fruit compote (pages 98–101) or fresh fruit, if desired.

Muesli is similar to overnight oats, but even more convenient, batch-able, and even gift-able! Feel free to swap out the pecans and raisins for an equal amount of any other nuts and dried fruit that you like. (See page 70 for sleep-supporting options.)

In a large bowl, stir together the oats, buckwheat flakes, pecans, raisins, maple sugar, chia, flaxseed, cinnamon, and salt. Transfer to an airtight jar and store in a cool, dark place for up to 2 months.

Overnight Oats
with Ginger, Winter Compote, and Walnuts

Serves 2	Total Time: 5 min., plus 8 hr. in the fridge

½ cup yogurt

1 Tbsp. honey or maple syrup

1 tsp. finely grated fresh ginger
or ¼ tsp. ground ginger

¼ tsp. ground turmeric

¼ tsp. vanilla extract

Pinch of kosher salt and
freshly ground black pepper

1 cup rolled (old-fashioned) oats

¼ cup Winter Compote
(page 100)

¼ cup coarsely chopped walnuts

Turmeric is an antioxidant
and it has been shown to help
mice get to sleep faster and to
increase their non–rapid eye
movement sleep. As a spice, it's
also a valuable addition to both
sweet and savory preparations
for its mild and earthy flavor
and sunny golden hue.

This sweet and gingery breakfast cereal can be enjoyed right from the fridge or zapped in the microwave for a quick morning meal. If your mornings are typically rushed (and whose aren't?), you can eliminate the last-minute prep work by batching this recipe out into single-portion plastic containers or jars. Oats contain loads of heart-healthy fiber and sleep-supporting tryptophan, while a scoop of fruit compote and a sprinkle of crunchy walnuts round out the dish with omega-3 fatty acids, melatonin, and serotonin. Feel free to swap out the Winter Compote for either of the other fruit compotes in this book (pages 98 and 101), a few Roasted Figs (page 243), or even store-bought fig jam.

1. In a 16-ounce jar, stir together the yogurt, honey, ginger, turmeric, vanilla, salt, pepper, and ¾ cup of water. Stir in the oats to thoroughly moisten, then cover tightly and refrigerate for at least 8 and up to 48 hours.

2. When you are ready to serve, spoon the oats into 2 bowls, top with Winter Compote and chopped walnuts, and serve.

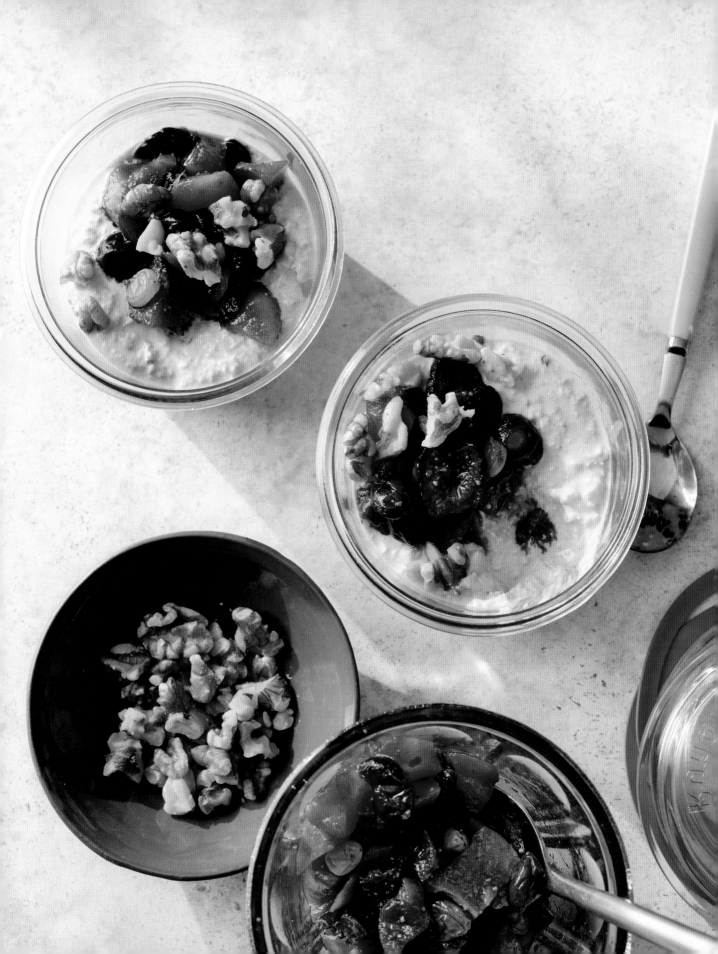

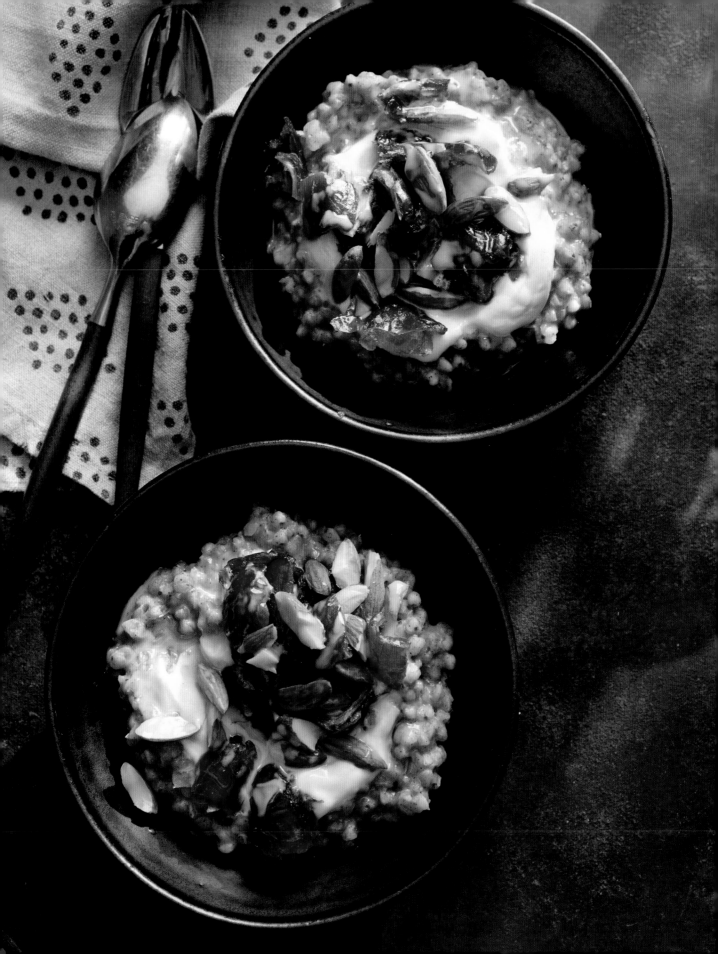

Spiced Buckwheat Porridge
with Dates, Tahini, and Greek Yogurt

Serves 2

Total Time: 20 min.

½ cup buckwheat groats

¼ tsp. ground cardamom

¼ tsp. ground cinnamon

Pinch kosher salt

½ cup milk

1 Tbsp. tahini

10 medium dates, pitted and torn into bite-sized pieces

¼ cup Greek yogurt

2 Tbsp. coarsely chopped almonds or 2 tsp. sesame seeds, for sprinkling

1 Tbsp. honey, maple syrup, or date molasses, for drizzling

Buckwheat groats, also known as kasha, are the hulled seeds of the buckwheat plant. (Buckwheat flour is simply finely milled buckwheat groats.) Like other whole grains, buckwheat is a great source of protein, tryptophan, and fiber, and it is also particularly high in a variety of other vitamins and minerals, including sleep-supporting zinc and magnesium. Buckwheat groats work nicely in both sweet and savory recipes and we especially like that they cook much more quickly than other whole grains like brown rice.

This warm and satisfying breakfast cereal is packed with protein and dietary fiber to keep you energized and sated all morning long. If you don't care for dates (like Marie-Pierre's son!), feel free to swap them out for a sliced banana.

1. In a small pot with a tight-fitting lid, stir together the groats, cardamom, cinnamon, and salt. Stir in ¾ cup cold water and the milk, then bring to a boil over medium-high heat. Lower the heat to maintain a simmer and cook, stirring occasionally, until the groats are soft, have almost completely absorbed their cooking liquid, but are not quite dry, 15–20 minutes.

2. Remove from heat and divide the porridge between 2 cereal bowls. Top with the tahini, dates, and Greek yogurt, sprinkle with almonds, drizzle with honey, and serve hot.

Banana-Berry Smoothie Bowl
with Chia and Granola

Serves 4 | Total Time: 10 min.

¼ cup rolled
(old-fashioned) oats

2 Tbsp. chia seeds,
plus more for garnish

½ cup milk or oat milk

2 cups mixed frozen berries

1 cup frozen pineapple chunks

2 medium bananas,
thinly sliced, divided

½ cup Greek yogurt

2 Tbsp. plus 2 tsp.
maple syrup, divided

2 Tbsp. almond butter
or sunflower butter

1 cup mixed fresh berries

½ cup granola

Time-Saving Tip: Leftover smoothies may be frozen in ice cube trays and reblended for last-minute weekday breakfasts and snacks.

This spoon-able riff on the Restful Smoothie (page 268) is designed for folks who prefer a bit more "chew" in the mornings. We love to top this dish with one of our own homemade granolas (pages 146–147), but all-natural store-bought versions work great, too.

1. In a blender, combine the oats, chia seeds, and milk and allow to soak until the oats are softened and the chia has gelled, about 5 minutes.

2. Add the frozen berries, pineapple, 1 of the bananas, the yogurt, 2 tablespoons of maple syrup, and the almond butter and blend until very smooth.

3. Assemble the bowls: Divide the smoothie mixture among 4 cereal bowls. Top with the remaining banana slices, fresh berries, and granola. Drizzle each serving with ½ teaspoon of maple syrup and garnish with a pinch of chia seeds. Serve immediately.

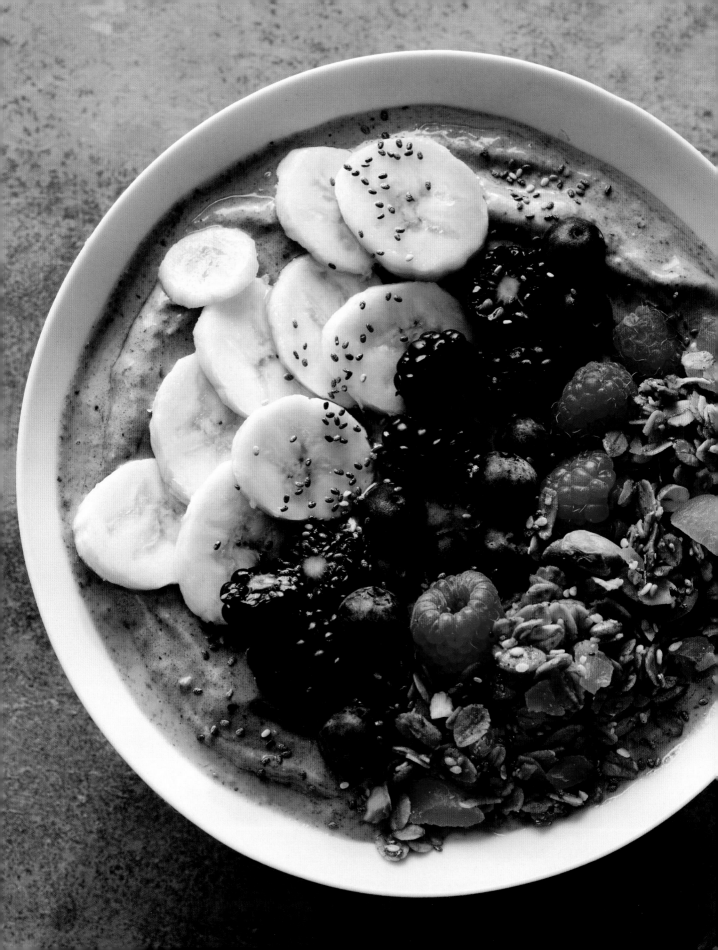

Muffin-Tin Quiche
with Salmon, Goat Cheese, and Spinach

Serves 6–12	Total Time: 1 hr.

½ lb. salmon fillet, skin removed (or substitute leftover cooked fish or poultry)

Kosher salt and freshly ground black pepper

Nonstick baking spray

2 cups baby spinach, lightly packed

Four 13- by 18-in. sheets phyllo dough

2 Tbsp. olive oil

4 large eggs

⅓ cup milk

1 tsp. Herbes Salées (page 117) (or substitute 1 Tbsp. finely chopped parsley mixed with ¼ tsp. kosher salt)

2 oz. fresh goat cheese (56 g)

These no-rolling-pin-required mini quiches look fancy, but they're actually quite simple to prepare. They're a great use for leftover salmon, but you can also swap in an equal amount of just about any other leftover cooked protein you have in the fridge—shredded chicken and turkey both work well, and shellfish like crab, lobster, or shrimp take the recipe to a whole new level. If you're using a leftover cooked protein, just preheat the oven and skip right to step 3.

If you do not like goat cheese, swap in strained ricotta or feta—if using the latter, you'll want to adjust the salt level accordingly. While these quiches are at their best fresh out of the oven, they also hold up well as a portable picnic lunch.

1. Position a rack in the center of the oven and preheat it to 350°F.

2. Season the salmon lightly with salt and black pepper. Grease a baking sheet or oven-safe skillet with nonstick baking spray, place the salmon on it, then bake until the fish is just barely cooked through, about 10 minutes. Remove from the oven and set aside to cool to room temperature. Increase the temperature to 375°F.

3. In a microwave-safe bowl, combine the spinach, a pinch of salt, and 1 tablespoon of water. Cover with plastic wrap or a lid, then microwave at full power until the greens are fully wilted and bright green, 1–2 minutes. (Alternatively, blanch the greens for 1 minute in a large pot of lightly salted water, then strain.) Set the spinach aside to cool to room temperature, then squeeze out as much moisture as possible and finely chop.

4. Meanwhile, make the phyllo shells: Lightly grease a standard muffin tin with nonstick baking spray. Lay 1 sheet of phyllo on a clean, dry work surface. (Keep the remaining phyllo covered with a sheet of plastic wrap or a damp towel to prevent it from cracking while you work.) Using a pastry brush, brush the first sheet lightly with olive oil, then top with a second layer of phyllo. Repeat with 2 more sheets to make a stack of 4, then, using a sharp knife, cut the stack into twelve 4-inch squares. Nestle the squares into the muffin tin and bake until the phyllo cups are lightly golden and crisp, 5–7 minutes. Set aside to cool slightly and increase the temperature to 400°F.

5. Using a fork, break the salmon into bite-sized pieces. In a small bowl, whisk together the eggs, milk, and Herbes Salées. Divide the salmon and spinach among the cups, followed by the egg mixture. Top each cup with some of the goat cheese, then bake until set, lightly puffed, and golden, 12–15 minutes. Cool slightly in the muffin tin, then use a thin knife or offset spatula to pop the quiches out onto a wire cooling rack. Serve warm or at room temperature; transfer leftovers to an airtight container and store in the fridge for up to 3 days.

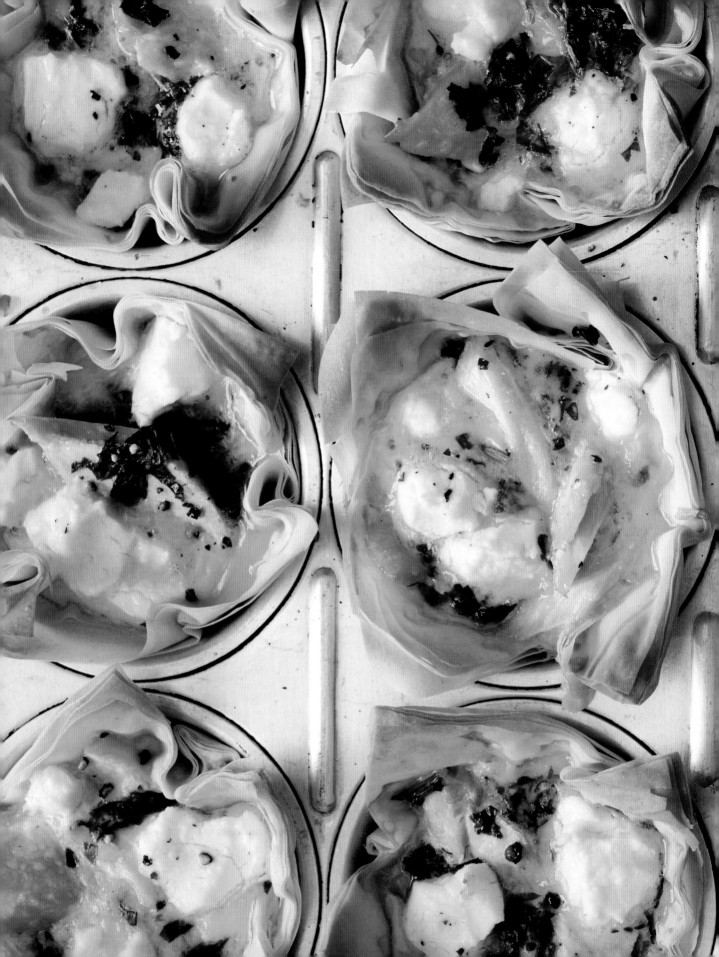

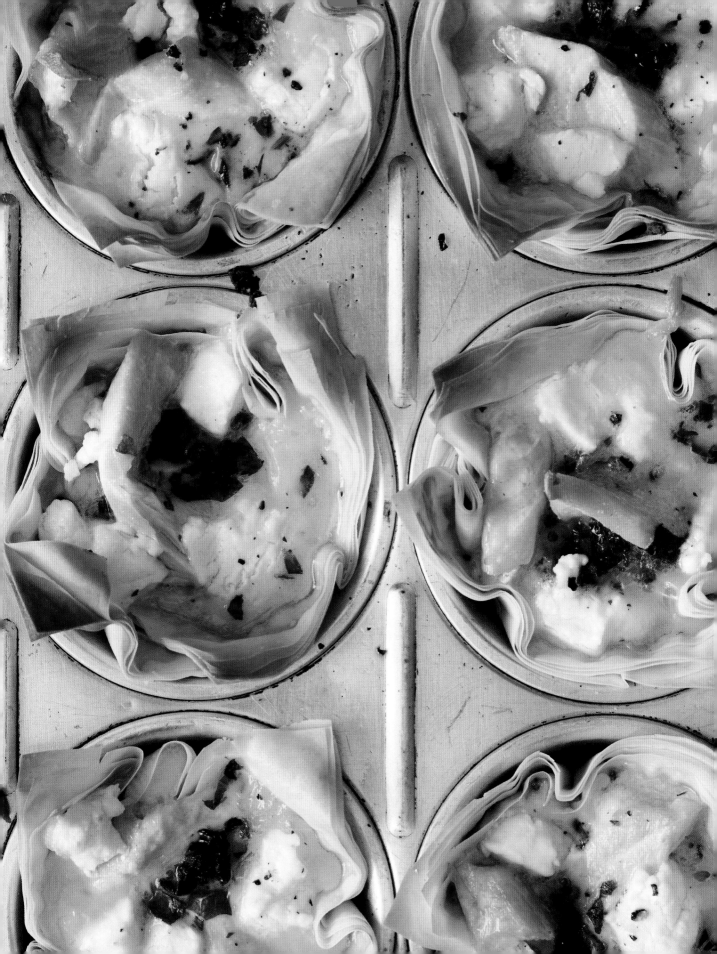

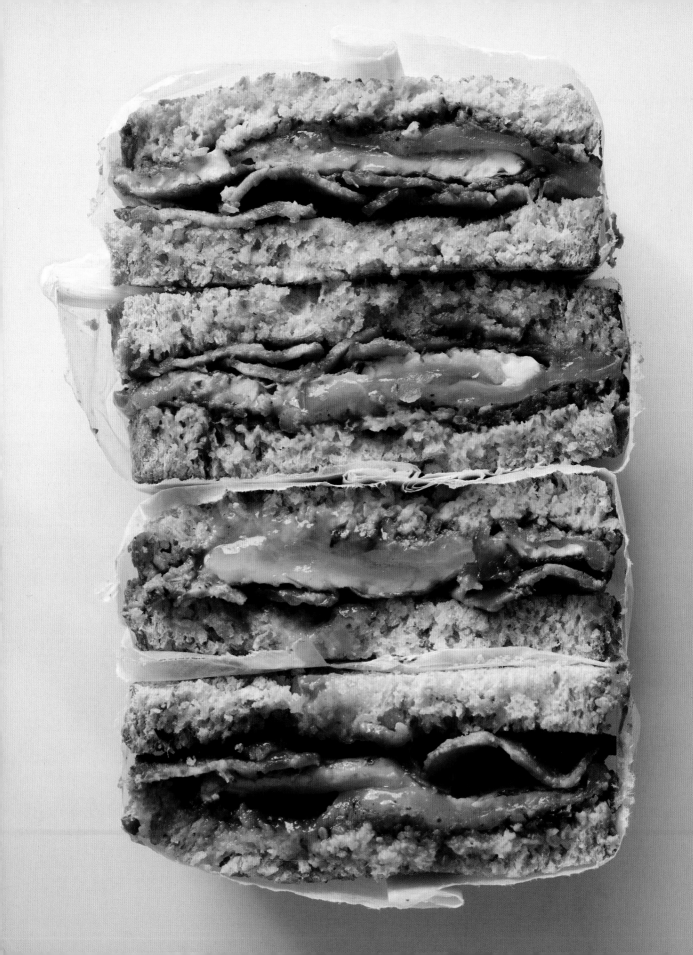

In-a-Hurry Egg-and-Cheese
with Salsa Roja

Serves 2 | Total Time: 15 min.

Nonstick cooking spray or olive oil

2 slices turkey bacon, halved crosswise

2 large eggs

Freshly ground black pepper

2 slices cheddar cheese

Four ½-in. slices Sesame-Sunflower Oat Bread (page 112), toasted

¼ cup Salsa Roja (page 124)

This protein- and tryptophan-rich sando comes together quickly and is perfect for grabbing on-the-go. We love to use our own homemade sandwich bread and a generous smear of melatonin-rich Salsa Roja, but any good-quality whole grain loaf and store-bought salsa are just fine.

1. Lightly oil a cast-iron or nonstick skillet with nonstick cooking spray and set it over medium-high heat. When the skillet begins to smoke, add the turkey bacon and cook, turning once, until crispy, 3–4 minutes. Transfer the bacon to a plate and set aside.

2. Return the skillet to medium-high heat and crack in the eggs; sprinkle with black pepper, cover, and cook until the whites are set, about 2 minutes. Flip the eggs (an offset spatula is helpful for this) and top each with a slice of cheese. Cover, lower the heat to low, and continue cooking until the cheese is melted and the yolk is cooked to your desired doneness, 2–3 minutes for a jammy consistency.

3. Uncover the skillet and transfer the eggs to 2 of the toast slices. Top with the reserved bacon, the Salsa Roja, and the remaining toast slices. Serve immediately or wrap the sandwiches in parchment paper to take to-go.

Sleep-Better Egg Toast
with Goat Cheese, Lemon, and Greens

Serves 1	Total Time: 10 min.

One ½-in. slice
Sesame-Sunflower
Oat Bread (page 112)
or other whole grain
sandwich bread, toasted

1 Tbsp. fresh goat cheese

2 tsp. extra-virgin olive oil

1 medium garlic clove,
thinly sliced

2 cups mixed baby greens

Kosher salt and freshly
ground black pepper

1 large egg

½ tsp. finely grated lemon zest

Fresh lemon juice

Pinch of crushed red
chile flakes (optional)

It's easy to forget about vegetables in the morning, when mealtime is so often dominated by processed meats, sugar bombs, and other refined carbs. That's why we love this quick and nutritious breakfast. Prewashed, mixed baby greens make easy work of sneaking nutrient-rich, sleep-supporting veggies into your morning routine, and this single-serve dish is as scalable as your toaster and largest skillet allows. We use our own Sesame-Sunflower Oat loaf here, but any store-bought whole grain bread will get the job done.

1. Spread the goat cheese over the toast and set aside on a plate.

2. Add the oil to a well-seasoned cast-iron or nonstick skillet over medium heat; when the oil begins to shimmer, add the garlic and cook, stirring frequently, until soft and fragrant, 1–2 minutes. Add the greens, 1 tablespoon of water, and a pinch of salt and cook, stirring occasionally, just until wilted, about 2 minutes.

3. Using tongs or a fork, transfer the greens to the toast, leaving the skillet over medium heat. Crack the egg into the skillet, season lightly with salt and black pepper, turn the heat down to low, and cook until the white is set and the yolk has reached the desired doneness (about 5 minutes for a runny yolk). Slide the sunny-side up egg atop the greens, garnish with lemon zest, a squeeze of fresh lemon juice, and crushed red chile flakes, if using, and serve hot.

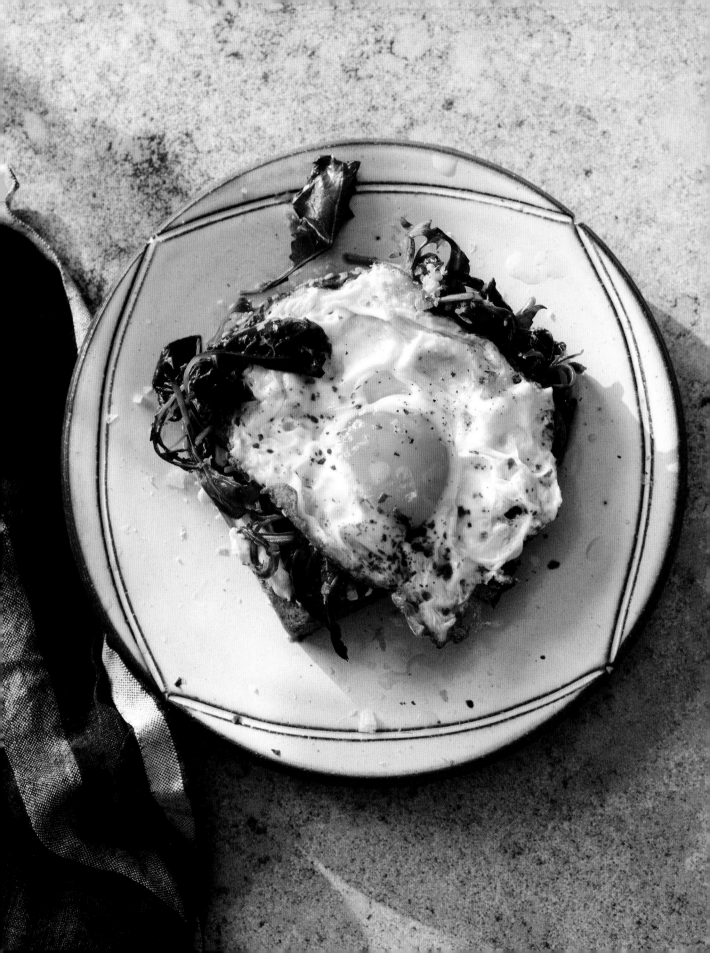

Sleepy Seeded Apricot-Pistachio Granola

Makes 4 cups

Total Time: 40 min.

2 cups rolled
(old-fashioned) oats

2 Tbsp. chia seeds

¼ cup extra-virgin olive oil,
plus more for greasing

⅓ cup honey or maple syrup

½ cup pumpkin seeds

3 Tbsp. sesame seeds

1 tsp. ground cinnamon

½ tsp. ground cardamom
(optional)

¾ cup chopped dried apricots

½ cup roasted pistachios,
coarsely chopped

½ tsp. flaky sea salt

Warming sesame seeds and spices in olive oil before mixing draws the natural oils in those ingredients out, resulting in a more fragrant and flavorful granola. Set a timer, stay in the kitchen, and keep an eye on the oven while this cereal bakes—depending on the heft of your baking sheet, granola can go from undercooked to burned very quickly. Stirring the oat mixture into the fruit and nuts helps the garnishes to cling to the still-sticky granola and prevents larger chunks from sinking to the bottom of the mix.

1. Position a rack in the center of the oven and preheat it to 325°F.

2. In a medium bowl, stir together the oats and chia seeds, then set aside. Line a large baking sheet with parchment paper, grease the paper lightly with olive oil, and set aside.

3. In a small pot, combine the honey, olive oil, pumpkin and sesame seeds, cinnamon, and cardamom, if using. Place the pot over medium-low heat and cook, stirring frequently, until the mixture is hot and very fragrant, 3–5 minutes. Remove from heat, then pour the liquid over the oat-chia mixture. Using a silicone spatula or large spoon, stir well until the oats are thoroughly coated.

4. Turn the oat mixture out onto the lined baking sheet and spread out to an even layer. Bake, stirring well every 5 minutes, until the granola is evenly browned and no longer sticky, 25–30 minutes. (The granola will seem wet while it is still hot, but if you transfer a small scoop from the baking sheet to a cool, dry plate, it should crisp quickly as it cools.)

5. Meanwhile, in a large bowl, stir together the apricots, pistachios, and sea salt. When the granola comes out of the oven, immediately fold up the edges of the parchment paper to carefully lift and transfer the hot cereal to the bowl. Stir to thoroughly combine, then pour the granola back onto the baking sheet to finish cooling. Once cool, the granola may be served immediately or transferred into an airtight jar and stored in a cool, dry place for up to 1 month.

Cocoa Nib Granola
with Candied Ginger, Cherries, and Almonds

Makes 4 cups

Total Time: 40 min.

¼ cup extra-virgin olive oil, plus more for greasing

2 cups rolled (old-fashioned) oats

⅓ cup honey or maple syrup

⅓ cup raw cacao nibs

3 Tbsp. sesame seeds

1 tsp. ground cinnamon

Pinch of ground nutmeg

¼ tsp. vanilla extract (optional)

¾ cup dried cherries

½ cup slivered almonds (optional)

¼ cup finely chopped candied ginger

½ tsp. flaky sea salt (optional)

Cacao nibs (aka cocoa nibs) are crumbled, fermented cacao beans, which are the main ingredient in chocolate. Candy manufacturers blend pulverized cacao nibs with sugars, emulsifiers, and other additives to make the sweet stuff we know and love. But the nibs are also delicious. We like to sprinkle them into homemade baked goods, where their nutty chocolate notes can be offset with a touch of sweetness.

With a sparkle of candied ginger, chocolatey cacao, and cheery dried tart cherries, this riff on our classic seeded granola makes an excellent special-occasion treat. Marie-Pierre also likes to make a big batch and package it up for holiday gifts.

1. Position a rack in the center of the oven and preheat it to 325°F. Line a large baking sheet with parchment, grease the paper lightly with olive oil, and set the pan aside.

2. Place the oats in a medium bowl. In a small pot, combine the honey, olive oil, cacao nibs, sesame seeds, cinnamon, and nutmeg. Cook over medium-low heat, stirring frequently, until the mixture is hot and very fragrant, 3–5 minutes. Remove from heat, stir in the vanilla, if using, then pour the liquid over the oats. Using a silicone spatula or large spoon, stir well until the oats are thoroughly coated.

3. Turn the oat mixture out onto the lined baking sheet and spread out to an even layer. Bake, stirring well every 5 minutes, until the granola is evenly browned and no longer sticky, 25–30 minutes. The granola will seem wet while it is still hot, but if you transfer a spoonful from the baking sheet to a cool, dry plate, it should crisp quickly as it cools.

4. Meanwhile, in a large bowl, stir together the dried cherries, almonds, if using, candied ginger, and the flaky sea salt. When the granola comes out of the oven, fold up the edges of the parchment paper to carefully lift and transfer the hot cereal to the bowl. Stir to thoroughly combine. Set aside to cool, then serve immediately or transfer to an airtight jar and store in a cool, dry place for up to 1 month.

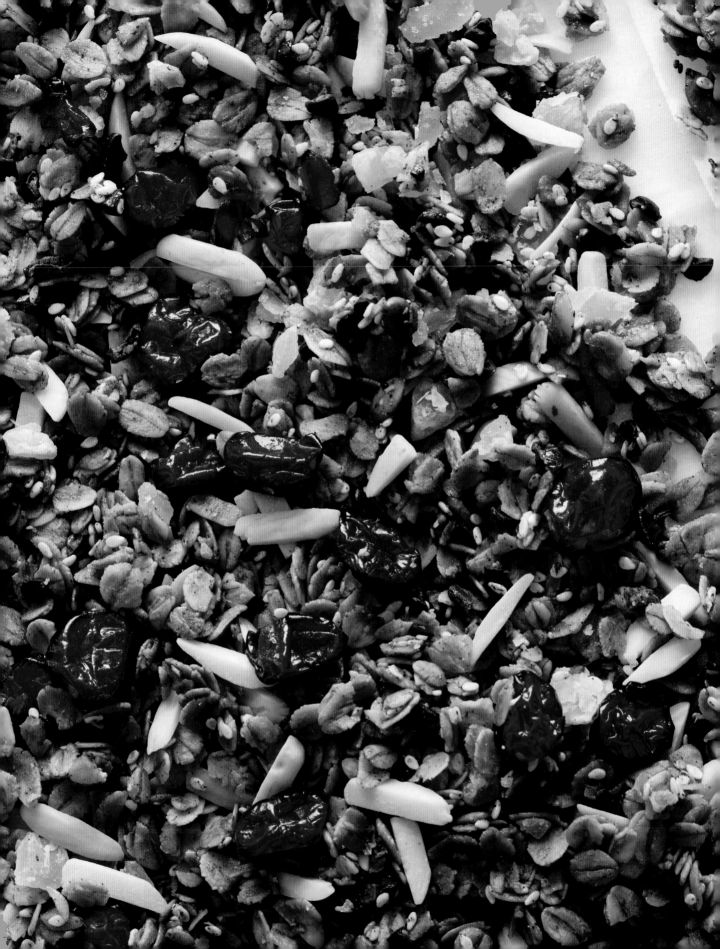

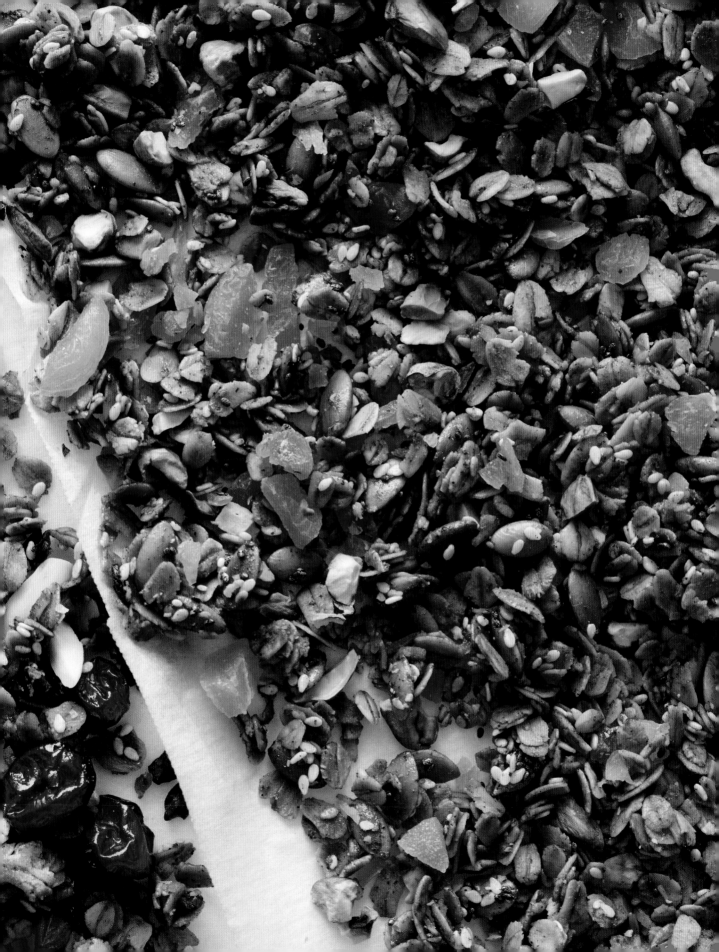

Make-Ahead Morning Muffins

Makes 12 muffins | Total Time: 25 min., plus time to soak the seeds

¼ cup sunflower seeds

¾ tsp. kosher salt, divided

½ cup Guinness or other stout beer

Nonstick baking spray (optional)

1½ cup (200 g) whole wheat flour

1 cup (125 g) all-purpose flour

2 tsp. baking powder

1½ tsp. cinnamon

1 large ripe banana or very ripe plantain, peeled and mashed (145 g)

1 large egg

½ cup buttermilk

⅓ cup olive oil

¼ cup molasses

½ cup bittersweet chocolate chips

We slipped as many sleep-supporting superfoods as possible into these nourishing little muffins. Taking the time to presoak the seeds the day before you bake prevents them from soaking up the moisture in the dough and ensures a moist and tender crumb. Look for all-natural, unsulfured molasses, which is better-suited to baking than blackstrap varieties.

1. The night before you plan to bake the muffins, soak the seeds: In a medium bowl, stir together the sunflower seeds, salt, and Guinness. Cover tightly and refrigerate for at least 4 and up to 24 hours.

2. Position a rack in the center of the oven and preheat it to 375°F. Lightly grease a 12-cup muffin tin with nonstick baking spray or fill the cups with paper liners. In a large bowl, whisk together the flours, baking powder, and cinnamon. In a medium bowl, whisk together the banana, egg, buttermilk, oil, and molasses. Stir in the reserved seeds and their soaking liquid and the chocolate chips, then, using a silicone spatula, fold the wet mixture into the dry ingredients until just combined.

3. Divide the batter evenly among the muffin tin cups and bake until the muffins are puffed and lightly browned and a toothpick inserted in the center comes out clean, 16–18 minutes. Serve warm, or cool completely, transfer to an airtight container, and store at room temperature for up to 3 days or in the freezer for up to 2 weeks.

Savory Whole Wheat Dutch Baby
with Turkey Bacon, Kale, Tomato Butter, and Eggs

Serves 6

Total Time: 25 min.

FOR THE DUTCH BABY

1 Tbsp. butter

1 Tbsp. olive oil

4 large eggs

¾ cup milk

½ cup whole wheat flour

¼ cup all-purpose flour

1 Tbsp. honey or maple syrup

½ tsp. smoked paprika (optional)

Pinch of kosher salt

FOR THE TOPPINGS

3 slices turkey bacon, halved crosswise

3 cups kale, rinsed, drained, stemmed, and cut into bite-sized pieces

1 tsp. olive oil

2 large eggs

Kosher salt and freshly ground black pepper

2 Tbsp. Tomato Butter (page 122)

A Dutch baby is a puffy, skillet-sized pancake and a dramatic (but very easy) canvas for all manner of sweet or savory breakfast items. Our version comes together quickly and easily. We swapped out some of the white flour for whole wheat for a kick of sleep-supporting fiber. A dollop of melatonin-rich beefsteak Tomato Butter makes these particular toppings shine. If you don't have a batch stashed in the fridge or freezer, swap it out for a handful of halved cherry tomatoes sautéed in a tablespoon of unsalted butter.

1. Position one rack in the top third of the oven and the other in the bottom third; preheat it to 450°F.

2. **Make the Dutch baby:** Place the butter and olive oil in a 10-inch cast-iron skillet and place the skillet on the bottom rack of the hot oven; allow the skillet to heat for 5 minutes.

3. Meanwhile, in a blender, combine the eggs, milk, flours, honey, paprika, and salt. Blend on high until the batter is completely smooth. (Alternatively, combine these ingredients in a medium bowl or pitcher and combine with an immersion blender.)

4. Carefully remove the hot skillet from the oven and swirl the butter and oil to coat the sides of the skillet. Carefully pour in the batter, then return the skillet to the bottom rack of the oven and bake until the pancake is puffed and evenly browned, 14–16 minutes.

—continued—

5. Meanwhile, make the toppings: Arrange the turkey bacon in a single layer on one side of a large rimmed baking sheet or oven-safe skillet; place the kale on the opposite side and toss with the olive oil. Place the baking sheet on the top oven rack, above the Dutch baby. Cook until both the kale and bacon are crispy, 10–15 minutes.

6. Crack the eggs into a small pot and beat with a fork; season lightly with salt and pepper and set the pot over medium heat. Cook, stirring frequently, until the eggs are just set, 1–3 minutes. Adjust the seasoning to taste, then remove from heat.

7. Remove the Dutch baby from the oven. Top with the crispy kale, soft-scrambled eggs, and turkey bacon. Dot with Tomato Butter, cut into slices, and serve hot.

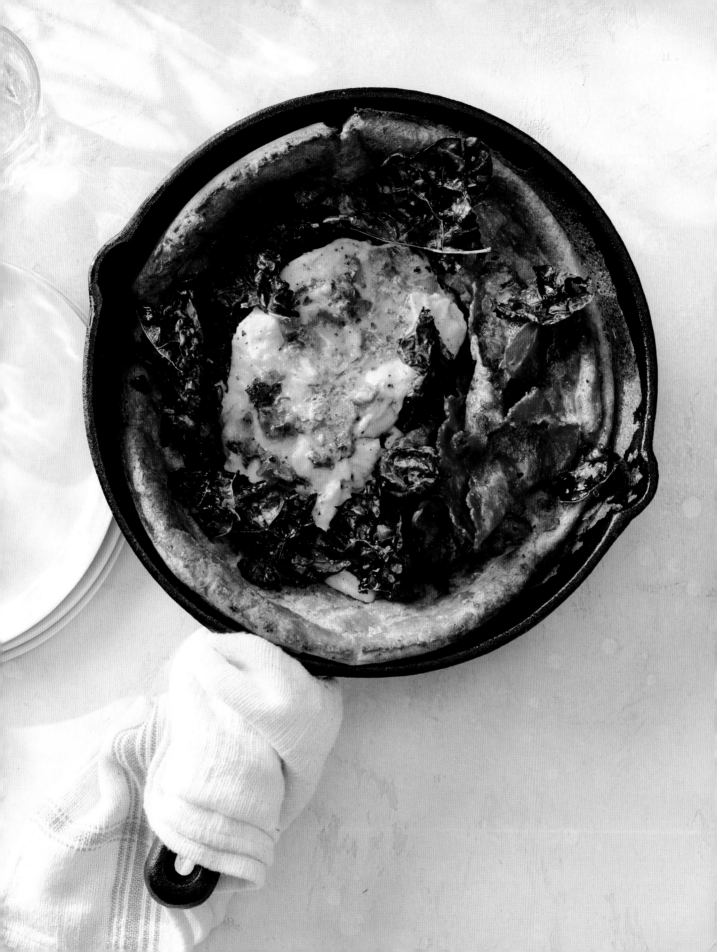

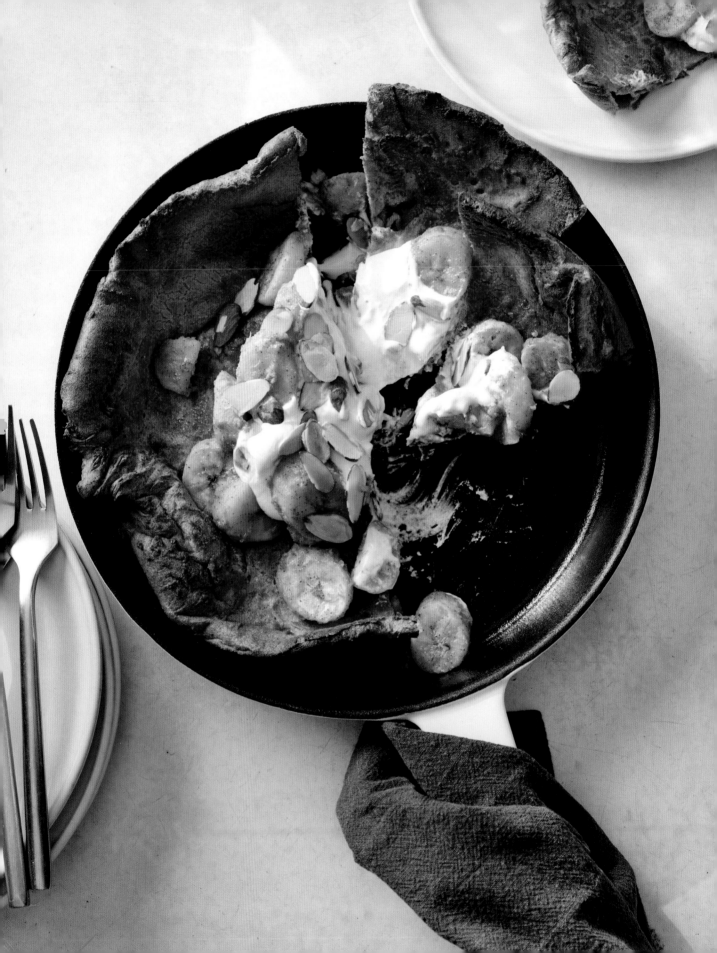

Sweet Whole Wheat Dutch Baby

with Honey-Butter Bananas, Greek Yogurt, and Almonds

Serves 6	Total Time: 20 min.

FOR THE DUTCH BABY

1 Tbsp. butter

1 Tbsp. olive oil

4 large eggs

¾ cup milk

½ cup whole wheat flour

¼ cup (32 g) all-purpose flour

1 Tbsp. honey or maple syrup

½ tsp. cinnamon

Pinch of kosher salt

FOR THE TOPPINGS

1 cup Honey-Butter
Bananas (page 103)

⅔ cup Greek yogurt

3 Tbsp. thinly sliced almonds

Our warm Honey Butter Bananas lend this sweet, family-sized breakfast a lovely tropical note, but feel free to swap in any fruit compote or fresh seasonal fruit you may have on hand.

1. Position a rack in the center of the oven and preheat it to 450°F.

2. **Make the Dutch baby:** Place the butter and olive oil in a 10-inch cast-iron skillet and place the skillet in the oven to preheat for 5 minutes.

3. Meanwhile, in a blender, combine the eggs, milk, flours, honey, cinnamon, and salt. Blend on high until the batter is completely smooth. (Alternatively, combine these ingredients in a medium bowl or pitcher and combine with an immersion blender.)

4. Remove the hot skillet from the oven and swirl the butter and oil to coat the edges of the skillet. Carefully pour in the batter, then bake until the pancake is puffed and evenly browned, 14–16 minutes.

5. **Add the toppings:** Remove the Dutch baby from the oven and top with the Honey-Butter Bananas, yogurt, and sliced almonds. Cut into slices and serve hot.

Family Brunch: Dry-Marinated Skirt Steak
with Fried Eggs, Pickled Mushrooms, and Grilled Tomatoes

Serves 4

Total Time: 35 min.

Savory Dry Rub (see opposite)

One ½-lb. skirt steak

2 large eggs

2 Tbsp. milk

1 tsp. Herbes Salées
(page 117) (or substitute
kosher salt to taste)

Kosher salt

2 large beefsteak tomatoes
(about 1 lb.), halved

4 slices Sesame-Sunflower
Oat Bread (page 112), toasted
and cut crosswise into points

1 cup Pickled Mushrooms,
drained (page 118)

Fresh cilantro or parsley
sprigs (optional)

We suggest seeking out meat
cut from grass-fed animals.
Grass-fed beef tends to be
lower in saturated fat and
higher in omega-3 fatty acids
than conventional grain-
finished types. Because of its
characteristic lack of fatty
marbling, grass-fed steaks can
become dry quickly, so don't
be tempted to walk away from
the stove and risk overcooking.
Skirt steak is an affordable,
comparatively lean, and quick-
cooking cut that takes well to a
flavorful dry marinade.

A heavy breakfast of steak and eggs is hardly the stuff of cardiologists' dreams—but there's something to be said for the high-quality protein (and high tryptophan levels) found in these tasty ingredients: steak, eggs, umami-rich pickled mushrooms, and grilled tomatoes. Always pair heavy proteins with high-fiber carbs and plenty of fresh sleep-supporting produce and make the most of an occasional indulgent brunch by taking the time to properly rest and slice pan-seared steaks and chops. Resting meat for a few minutes once it comes off the stove, then slicing it thinly across the grain, not only stretches a small amount of meat across several servings—it also ensures that each bite is at its most tender and juicy.

1. Rub the Savory Dry Rub all over the steak and set aside at room temperature. In a medium bowl, beat together the eggs, milk, and Herbes Salées and set aside.

2. Heat a large cast-iron or heavy nonstick skillet over medium-high heat. When the skillet is very hot, add the steak and cook until browned on one side, 2–3 minutes. Flip and continue cooking to your desired doneness, 2–4 minutes for medium-rare. Transfer the steak to a cutting board and set it aside to rest.

3. Lightly salt the cut sides of the tomatoes, then add them to the skillet, cut-side down. Cook until they are lightly charred on one side, 3–5 minutes. Using a thin metal spatula, flip and continue cooking until the tomato skins are lightly charred, 3–5 minutes more. Transfer the tomatoes to a warm platter and turn the heat to low. Wipe out the skillet (it doesn't need to be spotless). Add the egg mixture and cook, stirring continuously, until barely set, 1–3 minutes. Remove from heat and continue stirring until cooked through, about 30 seconds more. Transfer the eggs to the platter.

4. Using a sharp chef's knife angled on a diagonal against the grain, thinly slice the steak, then transfer the slices to the platter. Add the toast points and the Pickled Mushrooms, top with cilantro or parsley sprigs, if using, and serve hot.

Savory Dry Rub

½ tsp. freshly ground black pepper

½ tsp. ground cumin

¼ tsp. ground coriander

¼ tsp. garlic powder

¼ tsp. paprika

¼ tsp. kosher salt

In a small bowl, stir together the black pepper, cumin, coriander, garlic powder, paprika, and salt.

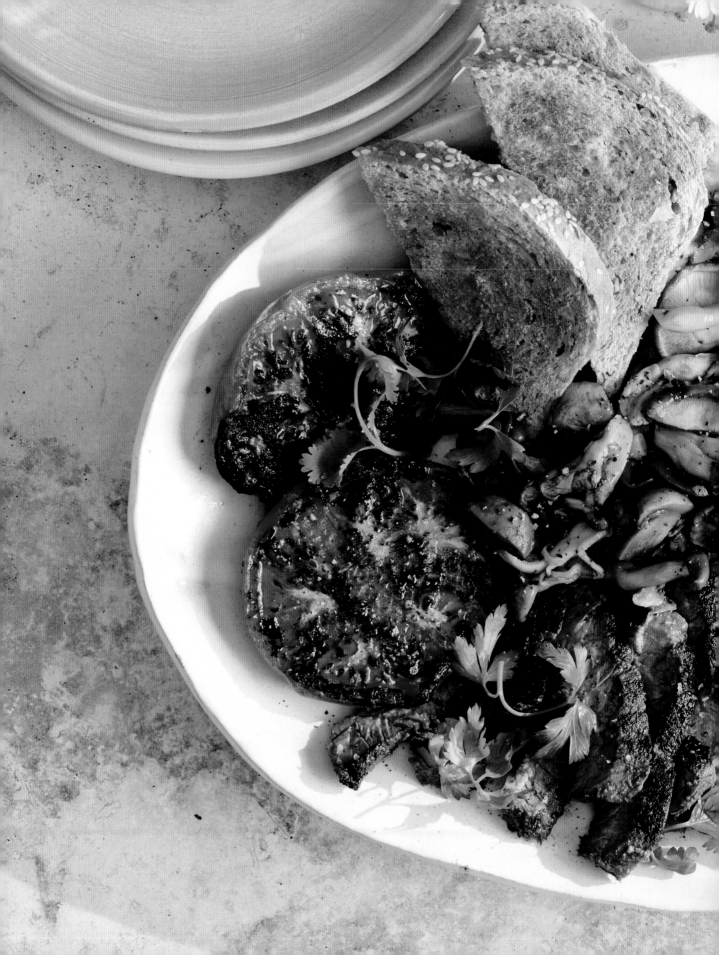

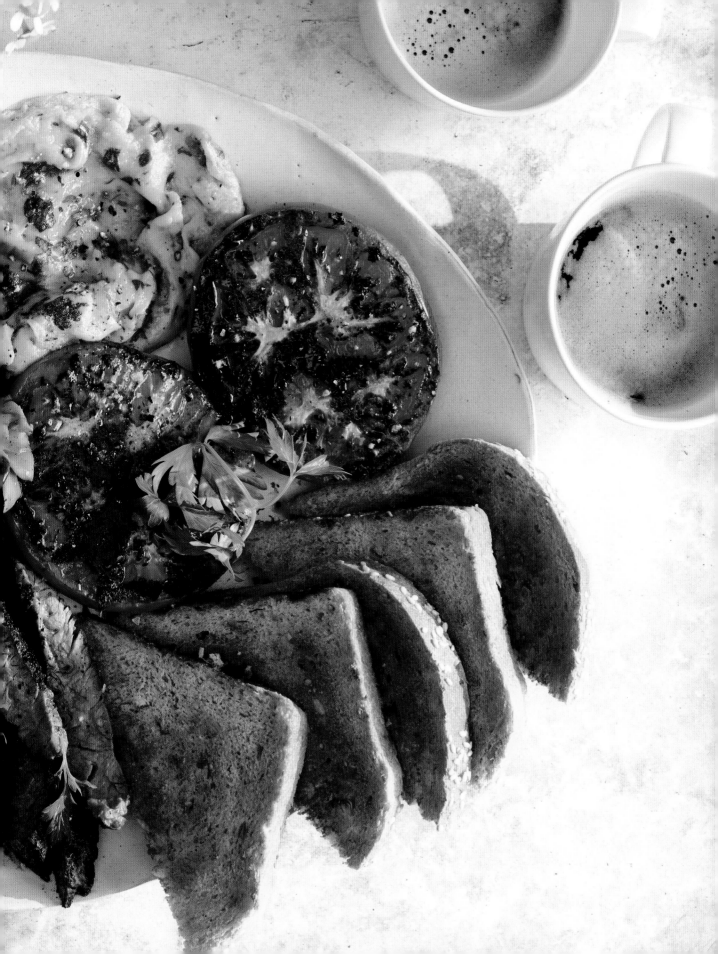

Whole Wheat Pancakes, Tropical Fruit Compote, and Sesame-Cashew Crunch

Serves 5

Total Time: 35 min.

1 cup milk

2 large eggs

3 Tbsp. maple syrup or honey

1 cup whole wheat flour

½ cup buckwheat flour

2 Tbsp. chia seeds

2 tsp. baking powder

½ tsp. fine sea salt

Nonstick baking spray

2½ cups Tropical Fruit Compote (page 101)

2½ cups Sesame-Cashew Crunch (page 104)

½ cup plus 2 Tbsp. Greek yogurt

Pro Tip: If you prefer waffles, whisk a tablespoon of cornstarch and 2 tablespoons of water into this pancake batter and cook on a waffle iron according to the manufacturer's instructions.

After decades of shrinking agricultural biodiversity, commercial farmers have begun to grow more heirloom crops. Today, farmers' markets and food co-ops can be a great source for a wide variety of lesser-known whole grain flours, including spelt, buckwheat, rye, and einkorn. If you're not quite sure what to do with these nutrient-rich ingredients, this basic pancake formula is a great starting point. Try swapping out the buckwheat for an equal portion of any other finely milled whole grain.

1. In a medium bowl, whisk together the milk, eggs, and maple syrup until combined. In a large bowl, combine the whole wheat and buckwheat flours, chia seeds, baking powder, and salt. Pour the wet ingredients into the flour mixture and whisk to combine.

2. Grease a medium nonstick or cast-iron skillet or a griddle with nonstick baking spray, then set over medium heat. When the skillet is hot, working in batches, use a ¼-cup measuring cup to add the batter to the skillet. Cook until bubbles form on the surface, 2–3 minutes. Flip the pancakes and continue cooking until evenly browned, 1–2 minutes more. Transfer to a warm plate and tent with aluminum foil while you continue cooking the rest of the batter.

3. Serve the pancakes warm, topped with Tropical Fruit Compote, Sesame-Cashew Crunch, and a dollop of yogurt.

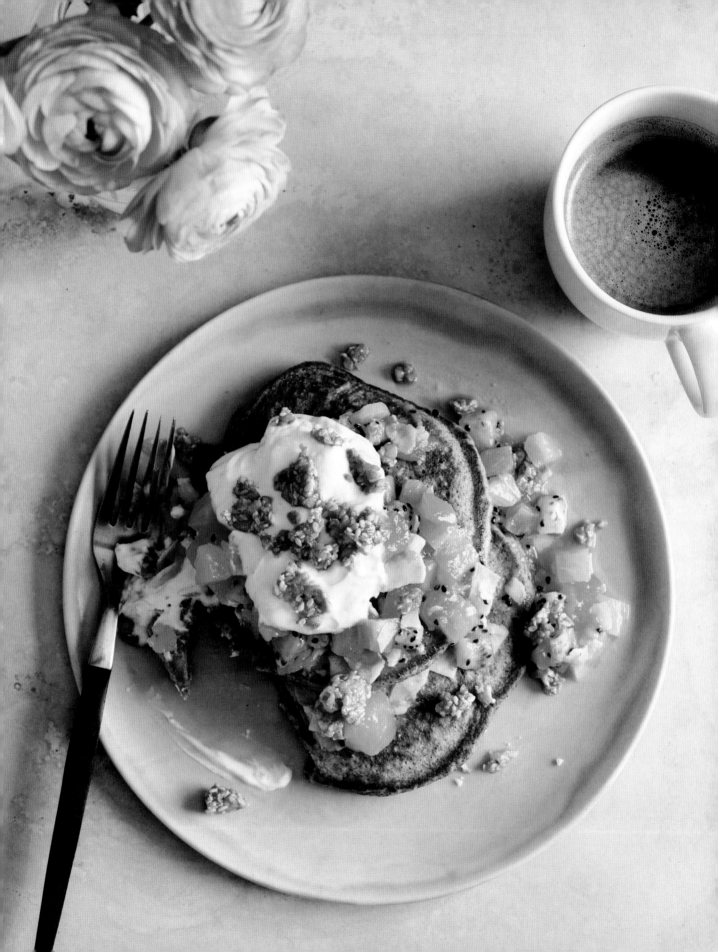

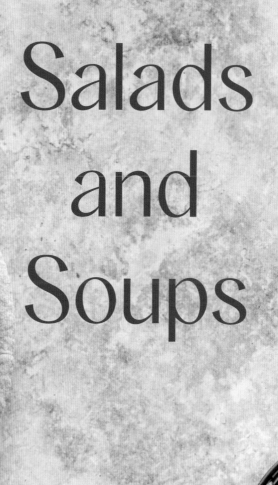

Salads
and
Soups

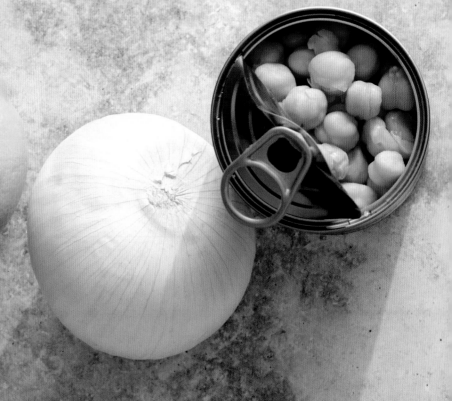

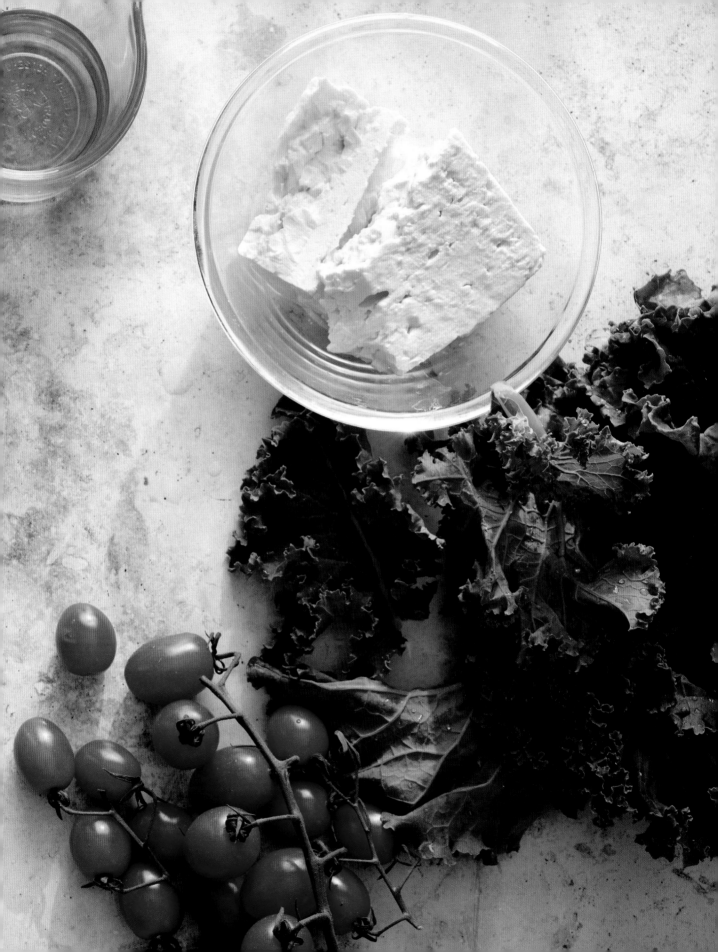

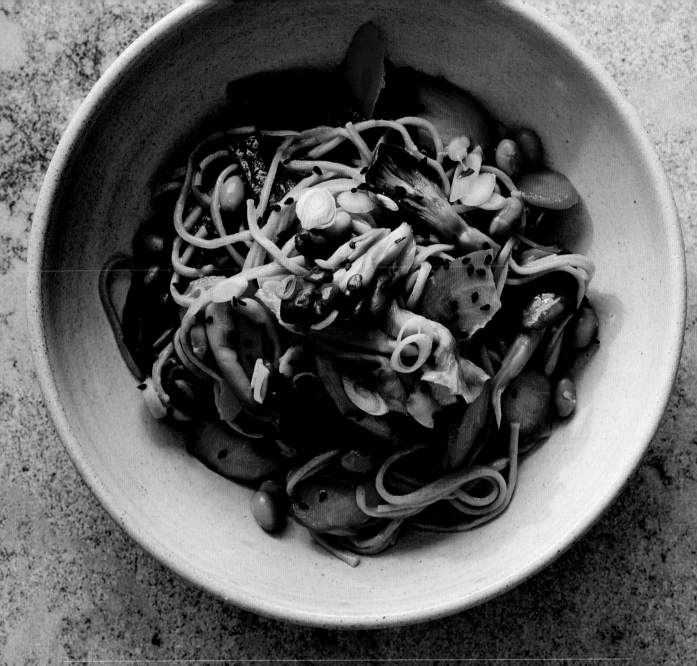

While we love the convenience of baby spinach in this salad, any tender greens will work just as well. We like to improvise with whatever is freshest at specialty grocers, farmers' markets, and our conventional grocery stores. Here are a few of our favorite Asian varieties, all of which can be swapped out seamlessly for other soft leafy greens like spinach or chard here and elsewhere in the book.

MORNING GLORY: Also known as hollow-heart vegetable, ong choy, and water spinach, these long, delicate greens have a mild flavor and tender-crisp hollow stalks.

CHOY SUM: This deep green leafy vegetable is a close relative to mustard greens and cabbage. Its thick stalks sometimes need a bit more time to cook than its delicate greens and edible yellow flowers. If the stems seem tough, separate, peel, and thinly slice them before cooking along with the leaves.

BOK CHOY: A type of Chinese cabbage and one of the best-known Asian greens, mild and crunchy bok choy is as easy to cook as it is to love. The faintly celery-like flavor of this widely loved green is especially tasty in soups, where its delicate greens turn soft and silky.

MIZUNA: This feathery vegetable is also known as Japanese mustard or spider mustard. With a delicate sweetness and very little bitterness, it may be pickled, enjoyed raw in salads, or lightly cooked in stir-fries or soups.

Chilled-Out Soba Salad
with Edamame and Sesame-Ginger Vinaigrette

Serves 4

Total Time: 25 min.

Kosher salt

3 cups baby spinach

3 medium carrots, peeled and very thinly sliced (1 cup)

1 cup shelled fresh or frozen edamame

One 8-oz. package dried buckwheat soba noodles

¼ cup Creamy Sesame-Ginger Vinaigrette (page 115)

¼ cup Pickled Mushrooms (page 118), drained, 1 Tbsp. brine reserved

2 Tbsp. thinly sliced scallions

1 tsp. sesame seeds

This cold and refreshing noodle salad is easy to prepare once you've stocked your fridge with some of our sleep-supporting pantry items. (And for this dish, store-bought Japanese-style pickles are a great substitute for our Pickled Mushrooms.) Seek out dried soba noodles that are made with 100 percent buckwheat flour. While the whole grain version is sometimes a little bit pricier than those made from a blend of wheat and buckwheat, the all-buckwheat noodles are preferable for their megaload of sleep-supporting tryptophan and fiber. As written, this recipe makes a refreshing side dish. Make it a light afternoon meal for two by topping each serving with a soft-boiled egg or a few ounces of crispy baked tofu.

1. Bring a large pot of lightly salted water to a boil over high heat. Meanwhile, place the spinach, carrots, and edamame in a colander in the sink. When the water is boiling, add the noodles and cook according to the package instructions. Once the noodles are just tender, drain them by pouring directly over the vegetables. Rinse well under plenty of cool, running water to remove any excess starch and stop the cooking.

2. Return the noodles and vegetables to the pot, add the dressing and the pickled mushroom brine, and toss to coat. Transfer to individual serving bowls, top each serving with pickled mushrooms, sliced scallions, and sesame seeds, and serve at room temperature.

Warm Pita Salad with Kale, Feta, Tomatoes, and Chickpeas

Serves 4

Total Time: 50 min.

8 oz. kale, leaves and stems separated

½ small white onion, sliced into ¼-in.-thick rings

¼ cup extra-virgin olive oil, divided

Kosher salt, to taste

1 cup cherry tomatoes, halved

One 15.5-oz. can chickpeas, rinsed and drained

Three 8-inch whole wheat pita breads

1–2 Tbsp. fresh lemon juice

Freshly ground black pepper

½ cup crumbled feta

1 tsp. ground sumac (optional)

Similar to Lebanese fattoush or Italian panzanella, this quick dish works equally well as a side dish or no-fuss one-pan supper. Sumac is a tart red berry that is dried, ground, and used as a spice. If you can't find it, an extra squeeze of lemon juice will do just fine.

1. Preheat the oven to 450°F. Line a large rimmed baking sheet with parchment or foil.

2. Slice the kale stems ¼ inch thick, then transfer to the baking sheet. Add the onion and 1 tablespoon of oil, season very lightly with salt, and toss to combine. Push the vegetables to one side of the sheet.

3. Tear the kale leaves into bite-sized pieces, then add them to a large bowl; add a tablespoon of oil and a pinch of salt and toss to combine. Transfer the greens to the center of the baking sheet. Next, in the same bowl, toss to combine the cherry tomatoes, chickpeas, another tablespoon of olive oil, and a pinch of salt. Transfer the mixture to the empty side of the baking sheet. Bake until the greens are crispy, the tomatoes and onions begin to brown, and the kale stem pieces are tender, 20–40 minutes.

4. Meanwhile, using a drizzle of the remaining olive oil, very lightly brush the pita on both sides. Place the breads on a second large baking sheet; bake until crispy, about 5 minutes. (If you don't have two baking sheets, you can also slide the pitas directly onto the oven rack as the vegetables cook.)

5. Set the bread aside until it is cool enough to handle, then tear into bite-sized pieces and place in the large bowl. When the vegetables come out of the oven, immediately scrape them into the bowl along with the pita. Drizzle in the remaining olive oil and 1 tablespoon of lemon juice and toss to combine. Season to taste with more lemon juice, salt, and black pepper and sprinkle over the feta and sumac, if using. Serve warm or at room temperature.

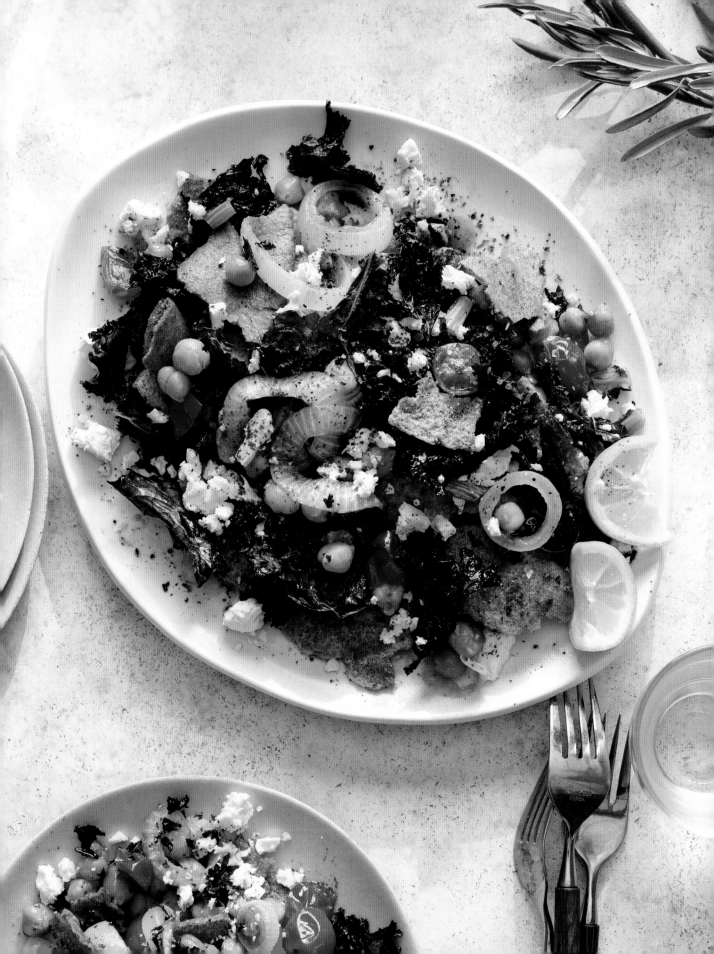

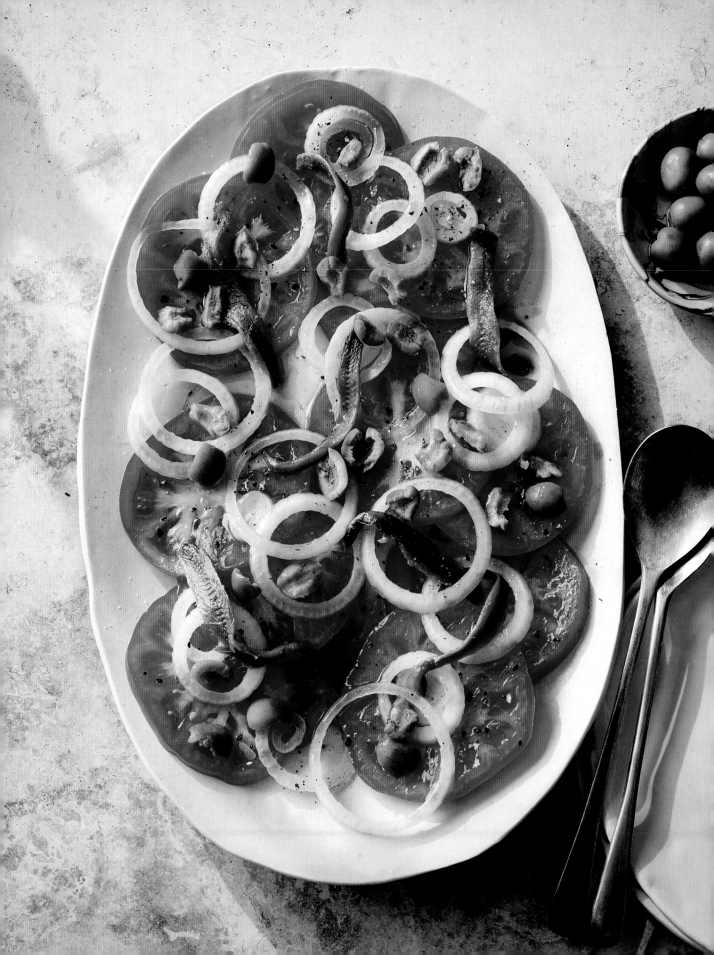

Tomato Salad
with Anchovy, Green Olives, and Onions

Serves 4–6

Total Time: 10 min.

3 medium beefsteak tomatoes (about 1½ lb.), sliced ¼ inch thick

1 small white onion, sliced ¼ inch thick

Pinch of kosher salt

Freshly ground black pepper

2 Tbsp. extra-virgin olive oil

1½ tsp. sherry vinegar

¼ cup pitted green olives, sliced

8 oil-packed anchovy fillets, drained (optional)

While high in salt, a few anchovies are a great way to get more brain-healthy omega-3 fatty acids into your diet. If the flavor of the whole fillets is too potent for your palate, mitigate their concentrated fishiness by mincing to a fine paste, then whisking into olive oil before drizzling over salads and roasted vegetables.

Late summer's best heirloom tomatoes don't just taste great—they're also a sleep-supporting ingredient. Beefsteak tomatoes in particular contain melatonin and serotonin. This Catalan-inspired salad calls for beefsteaks, which are available all year, although no doubt most delicious in the summer. Olives and anchovies add layers of savory flavor (as well as heart-healthy omega-3s), but if either are not to your taste, feel free to omit them. (For a vegan variation, capers may be substituted for the anchovies.) This dish makes a lovely, light lunch with crusty bread, or a zesty side dish with grilled meats or seafood.

On a large platter, arrange the tomato and onion slices. Sprinkle lightly with salt and black pepper, then drizzle over the olive oil and vinegar. Garnish with olives and anchovy fillets, if using, and serve.

Little Gem Salad, Blue Cheese Buttermilk, Tomatoes, and Garlic Croutons

| Serves 4 | Total Time: 15 min. |

FOR THE DRESSING

⅓ cup buttermilk

Pinch of garlic powder

Kosher salt and coarsely ground black pepper

1–2 tsp. fresh lemon juice

¼ cup blue cheese crumbles

FOR THE SALAD

4 heads little gem lettuce (or substitute small Romaine hearts, leaves separated)

½ lb. heirloom tomatoes, cored and cut into bite-sized pieces

Kosher salt and freshly ground black pepper

½ cup Garlic Croutons (see below)

We love the light buttermilk dressing in this sleep-healthy take on the classic wedge salad. Our homemade Sesame-Sunflower Oat Bread (page 112) makes excellent croutons, but any whole grain loaf—or even store-bought croutons—will work just fine. If you prefer a ranch-style dressing, omit the blue cheese and instead swirl in a pinch of onion powder and a handful of finely chopped fresh parsley, cilantro, or dill.

1. **Make the dressing:** In a small bowl, whisk together the buttermilk and garlic powder, then season to taste with salt, black pepper, and lemon juice. Stir in the blue cheese crumbles and set aside.

2. **Make the salad:** Arrange the lettuce and tomatoes on a large, chilled platter and season lightly with salt. Drizzle the dressing over the salad, then top with the croutons and more black pepper. Serve immediately.

Garlic Croutons

Preheat the oven to 375°F. In a large bowl, stir together **1 tablespoon olive oil**, **¼ teaspoon garlic powder**, and **a pinch of crushed red chile flakes** (optional). Season lightly with **fine sea salt** and **freshly ground black pepper**, then add **1 cup of whole grain bread cut into 1-inch cubes**. Toss to combine, then transfer to a large baking sheet, spread in an even layer, and bake, stirring occasionally, until crispy and browned all over, 12–15 minutes. Cool completely before using or before transferring to an airtight container. Homemade croutons keep well for up to 10 days.

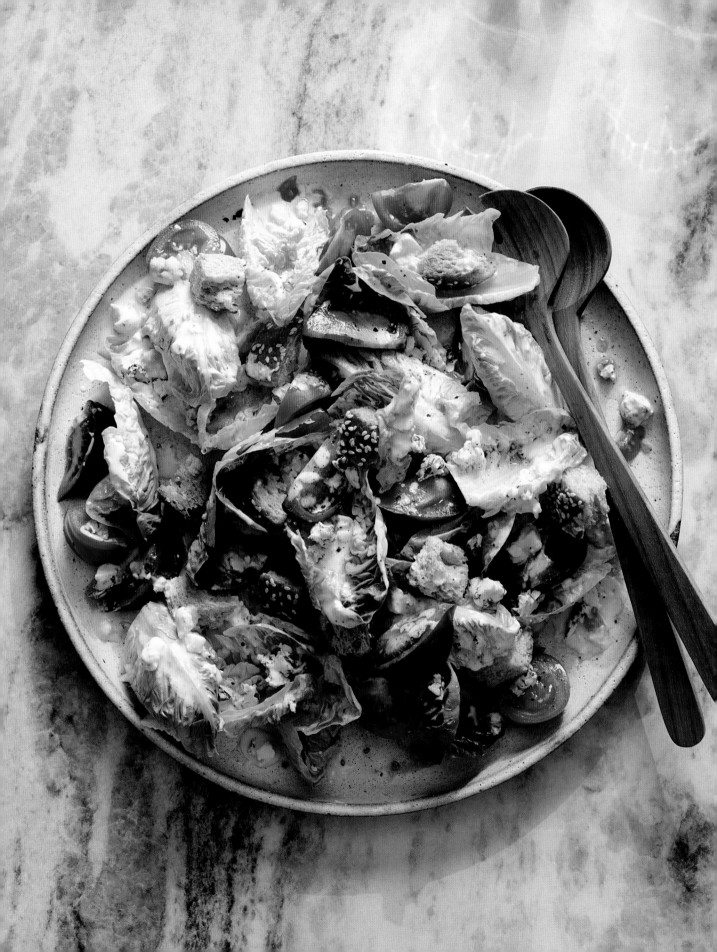

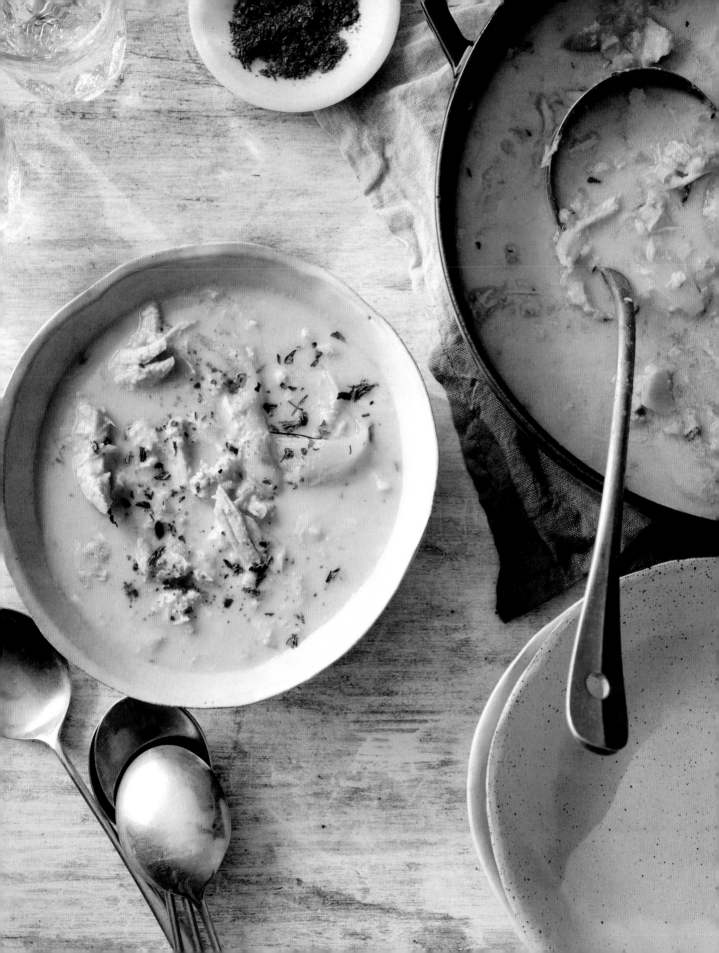

Creamy Lemon-Turkey Soup
with Barley and Mint

Serves 6

Total Time: 45 min.

1 Tbsp. extra-virgin olive oil

1 medium yellow onion,
finely chopped

4 medium garlic cloves,
lightly crushed and peeled

3 bay leaves

¾ cup pearl barley

9 cups homemade or low-
sodium chicken or turkey broth

5 large eggs

½ cup fresh lemon juice

2 Tbsp. finely grated lemon zest

2 tsp. dried mint, plus
more for topping

2 cups shredded cooked turkey

Kosher salt and freshly
ground black pepper

Crushed red chile flakes,
for garnish (optional)

Pro Tip: If you're meal prepping for the week and don't have leftover turkey on hand, buy a couple whole turkey legs, remove and discard the skin, and simmer the meat in a large pot of water with an onion, a celery stalk, and a carrot for an hour. Remove and discard the mushy vegetables, strain and reserve the broth for the soup, and, when cool enough to handle, shred the meat, discarding the bones.

Based on the homestyle egg-thickened Greek soup avgolemono, this nourishing bowl is our favorite use for leftover holiday turkey and a particularly soothing sick-day meal. Traditionally this dish is made with orzo or white rice, but we swapped those refined carbs out for pearl barley, which is higher in several sleep-supporting components, including fiber, tryptophan, gamma-aminobutyric acid (GABA), magnesium, vitamin B_6, and zinc.

1. In a medium pot, heat the oil over medium heat until it begins to shimmer. Add the onion, garlic, and bay leaves and cook, stirring frequently, until the onion is softened and translucent, 8–10 minutes. Add the barley and cook, stirring frequently, until it begins to smell lightly toasted, about 5 minutes. Add the broth, bring to a boil, then lower the heat to maintain a simmer and cook, stirring occasionally, until the barley is tender, 25–30 minutes.

2. In a small bowl, whisk together the eggs, lemon juice and zest, and the mint and set aside.

3. Stir the turkey into the soup and cook until heated through, about 2 minutes. Remove from heat and immediately and quickly whisk 2 cups of the broth into the lemon-egg mixture. Transfer the lemon-egg-broth mixture back into the pot, stirring continuously to prevent the eggs from seizing before they are completely incorporated. Return the pot to medium heat and cook, stirring and scraping the bottom of the pot continuously, until the liquid thickens, 4–6 minutes. (Don't let the mixture boil.) Remove from the heat and season to taste with salt and black pepper. To serve, divide the soup among bowls and top with more mint and black pepper and sprinkle with the chile flakes, if using.

Barley Salad

with Spinach, Feta, Pickled Mushrooms, and Walnuts

Serves 4

Total Time: 45 min.

Kosher salt

1 cup pearl barley

1 cup Pickled Mushrooms (page 118) plus ¼ cup reserved brine

2 Tbsp. extra-virgin olive oil

4 medium scallions, trimmed and thinly sliced

¼ tsp. ground coriander

3 cups baby spinach

Freshly ground black pepper

¾ cup crumbled feta

⅓ cup finely chopped fresh parsley

¼ cup coarsely chopped walnuts

Fresh herbs like cilantro, basil, and mint share many of the same nutritional benefits of the more expected leafy greens. This grain salad gets its freshness in part from a generous portion of parsley and scallions, which are treated here like salad vegetables rather than seasonings.

We like to serve this dish alongside grilled meat or fish. It also travels nicely and keeps well in the fridge, making it perfect for picnics, potlucks, and meal prepping. Make it a full meal by tossing in a cup of drained canned chickpeas or white beans. If you don't have time to make your own pickled mushrooms, store-bought ones are great in a pinch.

1. Bring a medium pot of lightly salted water to a boil over medium-high heat. Stir in the barley, lower the heat to medium, and cook, stirring occasionally, until the grains are tender, 25–30 minutes.

2. Meanwhile, in a large bowl, toss together the Pickled Mushrooms with their brine, the olive oil, scallions, and coriander; set aside.

3. When the barley is tender, stir in the spinach and continue cooking just until the leaves are wilted and bright green, 2–3 minutes. Remove from heat, strain, and then immediately transfer the hot barley-spinach mixture to the reserved mushroom-scallion dressing. Set aside, stirring occasionally, until cooled to room temperature, or transfer to an airtight container and refrigerate for up to 2 days.

4. Immediately before serving, season to taste with salt and black pepper, then gently fold in the feta, parsley, and walnuts.

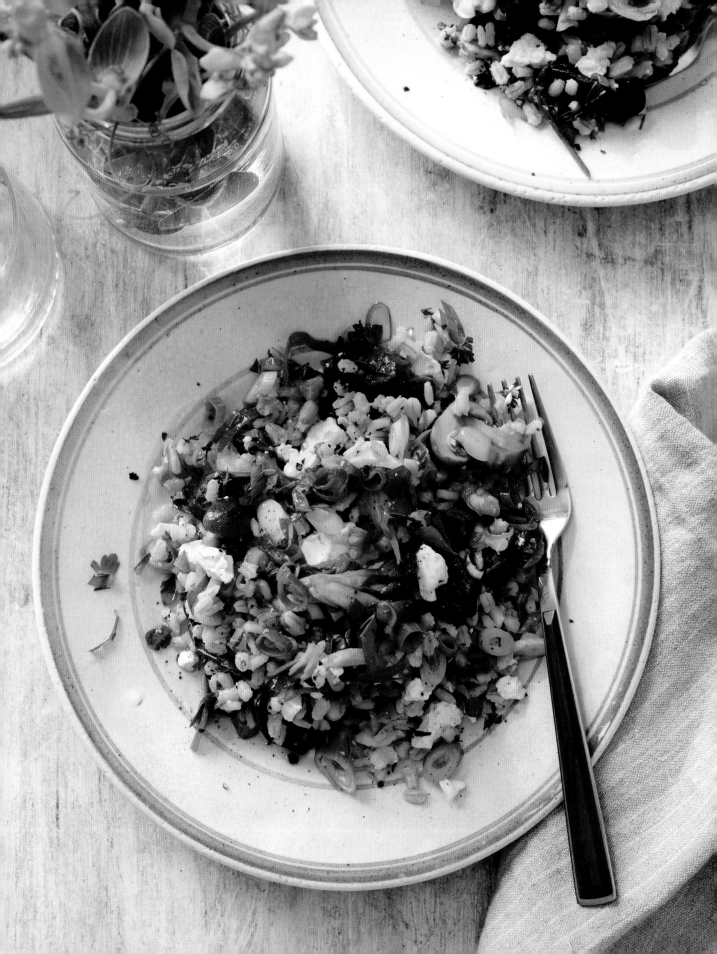

By weight, saffron—the stigmas of the *Crocus sativus* flower—is the world's most expensive spice, but just a pinch of this potent ingredient goes a long way toward enhancing both the flavor and color of a dish. In recent years, some researchers have also begun to explore saffron's potential effects on brain function and mental health, and there is some exciting evidence that suggests that consuming it may improve sleep quality by increasing melatonin levels. While much more research needs to be done before we can confidently point to saffron as an aid in managing sleep problems, there's certainly no harm in incorporating the ingredient into your cooking. We love it in seafood, chicken, and rice dishes, or even added to sweet foods like creamy pudding and hot tea. Like all premium products, saffron price and quality can vary substantially between sources, so we prefer to buy direct from single-origin, direct-to-consumer companies like Burlap & Barrel, Diaspora Co., and Moonflowers. Soaking the stigmas in hot water for a few minutes before using helps to draw out their deep golden color and distinctive fragrance.

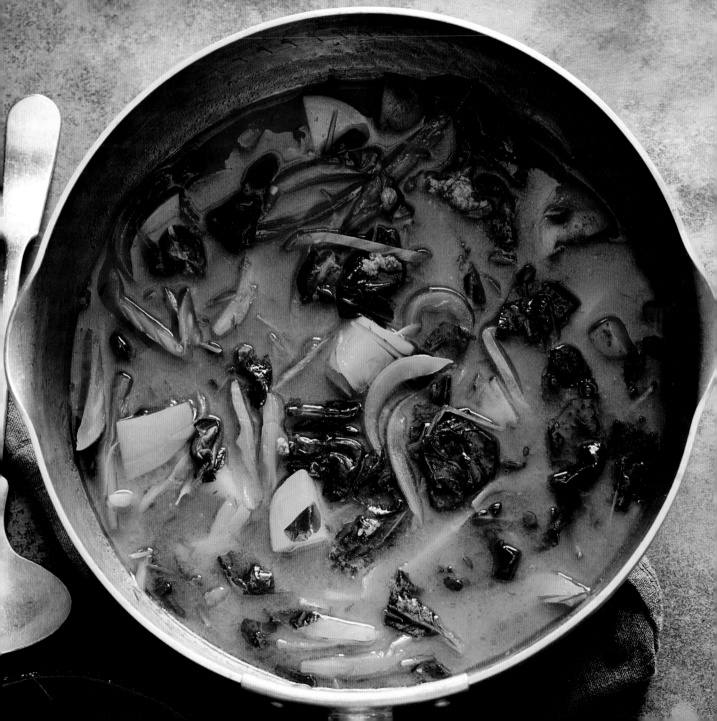

Smoky Oyster Chowder
with Saffron, Fennel, and Kale

Serves 3–4	Total Time: 35 min.

1 big pinch (about
20 threads) of saffron

1 Tbsp. extra-virgin olive oil

1 small yellow onion, thinly sliced

½ medium fennel bulb,
cored and thinly sliced

2 medium red or yellow
potatoes, cut in ½-in. cubes

Kosher salt and freshly
ground black pepper

1 tsp. smoked paprika

2 Tbsp. all-purpose flour

2 cups clam broth or fish stock

3 cups baby kale (or substitute
ordinary kale, stems removed
and discarded, leaves torn
into bite-sized pieces)

One 3.7-oz. can smoked oysters,
drained and coarsely chopped

Shellfish like oysters are an
excellent source of zinc, which
is involved in recovery, cell
growth, and immune function.
In a randomized controlled trial,
adults consuming a diet rich in
zinc from oysters took less time
to fall asleep and had better
sleep efficiency than those
given a placebo.

The aromatic broth for this quick, tryptophan-rich chowder is enriched with olive oil, smoked paprika, and saffron, while starchy red potatoes provide the carbs your brain needs to convert that important amino acid into serotonin and melatonin.

Good-quality tinned seafood is a convenient way to add a helping of lean protein and sleep-supporting nutrients to your diet in a hurry; in this recipe, smoked oysters, added at the last minute, lend depth of flavor and a whole day's worth of your body's nutrient requirements for zinc, as well as a welcome dose of B vitamins. A good handful of kale provides an extra hit of folate and B_6, while fennel and onion deliver plenty of flavor, fragrance, and fiber.

1. In a small bowl, combine the saffron and 1 tablespoon of hot water; set aside.

2. In a medium pot, heat the oil over medium heat until it begins to shimmer. Add the onion and fennel and cook, stirring frequently, until the onion is translucent but not yet colored, about 5 minutes. Add the potatoes, season lightly with salt, black pepper, and smoked paprika, and continue cooking, stirring occasionally, until the fennel is tender but still slightly crisp, about 5 minutes more. Sprinkle the flour over the vegetables and stir to coat, then slowly stir in the clam broth. Add the reserved saffron mixture and 2 cups of cool water, turn the heat up to medium-high, bring to a full boil, and cook for 1 minute. Lower the heat to maintain a simmer and continue cooking until the potatoes begin to soften, 10–15 minutes.

3. Add the kale and continue cooking until the greens are wilted and soft but still vibrant and the potatoes are tender, about 5 minutes. Remove from heat and stir in the chopped oysters. Season to taste with additional salt and pepper, ladle into soup bowls, and serve hot.

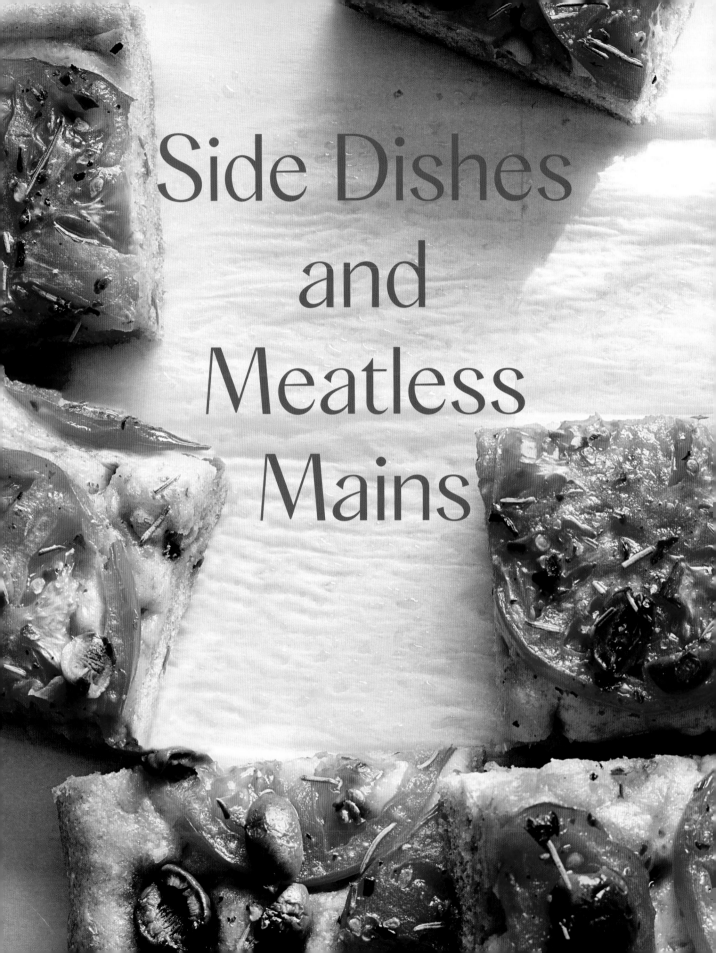

Side Dishes and Meatless Mains

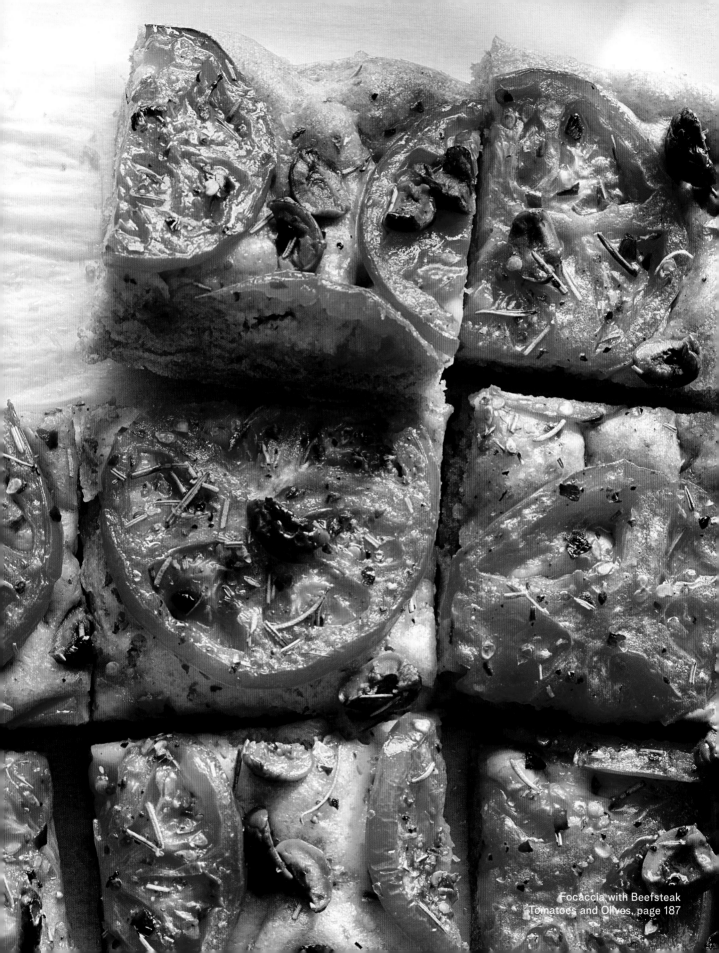

Focaccia with Beefsteak
Tomatoes and Olives, page 187

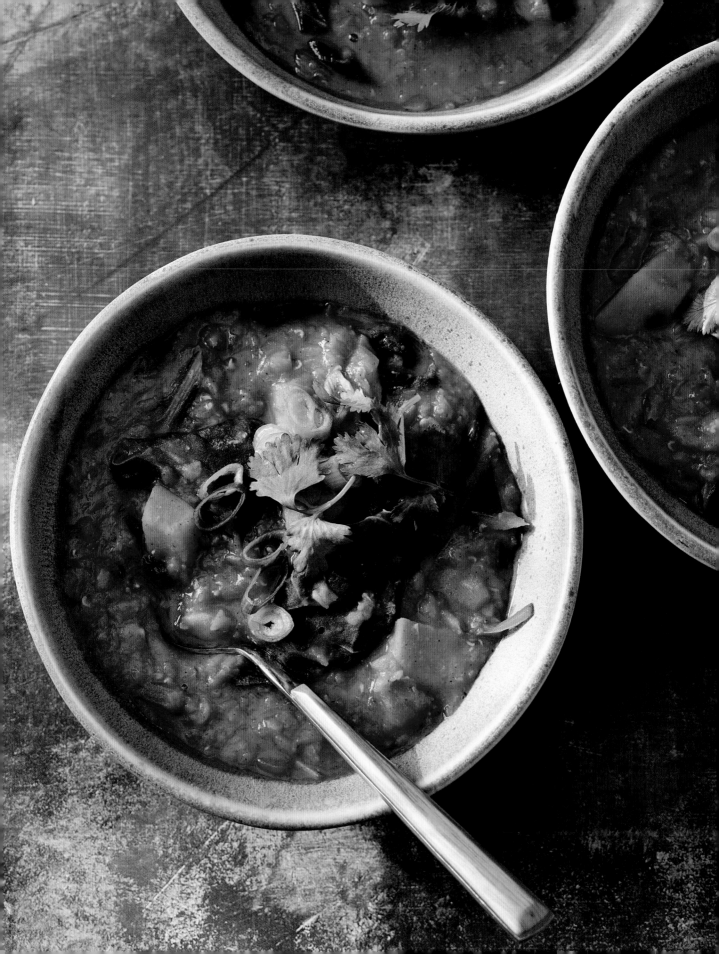

Spiced Red Lentils

with Coconut, Sweet Potato, and Greens

Serves 8–10	Total Time: 1 hr. 30 min.

1 bunch Swiss chard, trimmed

1 Tbsp. olive oil

1 medium sweet potato, peeled and cut in ½-in. cubes

Kosher salt

2 small onions, and finely chopped

1 large bell pepper, stemmed, seeded, and finely chopped

One 3-in. piece fresh ginger, finely chopped

6 medium garlic cloves, finely chopped

1 Tbsp. garam masala (or substitute curry powder)

½ tsp. turmeric

One 14½-oz. can crushed tomatoes

2 cups red lentils, rinsed and drained

3 cups vegetable or chicken broth (or substitute water)

One 14-oz. can lite coconut milk

Fresh cilantro sprigs and thinly sliced scallions, for garnish

Indian red chile powder or cayenne pepper (optional)

This economical, nutrient-dense, and entirely plant-based dish is one of our favorite meal-prep numbers: It keeps well for several days in the fridge or up to 3 months in the freezer. To make it a full meal, serve with a scoop of brown basmati rice or whole wheat naan, which you can usually find at the supermarket. Garam masala is a popular Indian spice blend readily available in well-stocked supermarkets and South Asian grocery stores, but if you can't find it or have run out, you may substitute curry powder. If spicy food causes you indigestion, leave out the chile powder, and if onions and garlic are an irritant, reduce the amount used, or omit them entirely as well. If you like, a pinch of asafetida may be added to the oil with the sweet potatoes to make up for the alliums' pungent note (see "Indigestion and Acid Reflux," page 56).

1. Separate the chard stalks and leaves; tear the leaves into bite-sized pieces; thinly slice the stalks on the diagonal. Set both aside.

2. In a large heavy pot, heat the oil over medium heat until it begins to shimmer. Add the sweet potato, season lightly with salt, and cook, stirring occasionally, until lightly browned, 5–6 minutes. Using a slotted spoon, transfer the sweet potato to a bowl and set aside.

3. Return the pot to medium heat and add the onions, bell pepper, and the reserved chard stalks. Season lightly with salt and cook, stirring frequently, until the vegetables begin to sweat and the onions are translucent, 3–4 minutes. Stir in the ginger, garlic, garam masala, and turmeric and cook until very fragrant, about 1 minute. Add the tomatoes and cook, stirring frequently, until the mixture looks dry and jammy, 2–3 minutes. Add the lentils, broth, and 1 cup of water, bring to a boil, then cover and lower the heat. Simmer, stirring occasionally, until the lentils are tender, 15–20 minutes.

Dried lentils are naturally high in protein and tryptophan, they contain melatonin, and they also cook much more quickly than dried beans, making them one of our star sleep-supporting pantry ingredients. These legumes sometimes pick up small pebbles and other debris during processing, so before you begin to cook, spread them out on a large rimmed baking sheet and pick out and discard anything that doesn't look like a lentil.

4. Uncover the pot, stir in the coconut milk and the reserved sweet potatoes, then increase the heat to medium. Bring to a simmer and cook, stirring frequently, until the lentils begin to dissolve and the sweet potatoes are very tender, about 15 minutes.

5. Add the chard leaves and continue cooking until they're wilted and tender, 6–8 minutes. Remove from heat, season to taste with more salt, then ladle into wide soup bowls. Garnish with cilantro sprigs and sliced scallions and a sprinkling of chile powder, if using. Serve hot.

Sopes

with Black Beans, Queso Fresco, and Curtido

Serves 2 for a full meal or
4–8 as a side dish

Total Time: 1 hr. 10 min.

FOR THE CABBAGE CURTIDO

2 cups thinly sliced
green cabbage

½ cup thinly sliced red cabbage

1½ cups thinly sliced red onions

½ cup thinly sliced radishes

½ cup thinly sliced carrots

1 cup red wine vinegar

¼ cup honey

1 Tbsp. kosher salt

1 serrano chile, stemmed
and thinly sliced

1 tsp. whole coriander seeds

—*ingredients continue*—

Masa harina is a whole grain corn flour used mainly for making tortillas, tamales, and other Latin American breads. The Maseca and Bob's Red Mill brands are widely available. Corn masa's rich flavor and hearty texture is perfect for these sopes—thick and toothsome corn cakes that can be crowned with any number of savory toppings. We've also included a method for making your own refried beans here, but you can also use a ready-made, canned version.

Kat learned to make curtido—a tart, slaw-like pickle used widely throughout Central America—from Honduran American baker and cookbook author Bryan Ford. The recipe below makes more than you'll need for the sopes; store leftover curtido in an airtight container in the fridge for up to a month and add it to egg sandwiches, tacos, grain bowls, or any dish that could benefit from a bit of zippy crunch. If you are prone to heartburn and sensitive to spicy foods, feel free to replace the onions with extra carrots and omit the chile.

1. **Make the cabbage curtido:** In a large bowl, toss together the green and red cabbage, onions, radishes, and carrots. In a small pot over medium heat, combine the vinegar, honey, salt, chile, and coriander. Bring to a simmer, then pour the liquid over the cabbage mixture and toss to coat. Cover and set aside to cool to room temperature or transfer to the fridge and store for up to 1 month.

—*continued*—

2 cups instant masa harina

½ tsp. kosher salt

½ tsp. baking powder

¼ cup plus 1 Tbsp. extra-virgin olive oil, divided

½ cup finely chopped yellow onion

2 garlic cloves, finely chopped

One 15.5-oz. can black beans, rinsed and drained

2 cups low-sodium chicken or mushroom stock

¾ cup crumbled queso fresco or shredded Monterey Jack

¼ cup Salsa Roja (p. 124) (or substitute a store-bought salsa)

Fresh cilantro sprigs, for garnish (optional)

2. **Make the sopes:** In a large bowl, whisk together the masa, salt, and baking powder, then whisk in ¼ cup of the olive oil and 1½ cups of warm water until a soft dough forms. Cover and set aside until the dough stiffens and cools to room temperature, about 30 minutes.

3. Meanwhile, make the refried beans. In a large skillet, heat the remaining oil over medium heat until it begins to shimmer. Add the onion and cook, stirring frequently, until translucent, 2–3 minutes. Add the garlic and continue cooking until very fragrant, about 1 minute more. Add the beans and ¼ cup of the stock and cook, scraping up any browned bits, until the mixture begins to bubble, about 5 minutes. Gradually ladle in the rest of the stock, about ¼ cup at a time, stirring occasionally and smashing the beans gently with a wooden spoon. Remove from heat, cover the pan, and set aside.

4. Heat a large, seasoned cast-iron or nonstick skillet or a griddle over medium-high heat. Turn the masa dough out onto a clean work surface and divide it into 8 even pieces. Flatten each piece into a 4-inch disk, then cook the disks in batches: Place in the hot skillet and cook until lightly browned, 3–4 minutes. Using a wide, thin spatula, flip the disks, then top each with about 3 tablespoons of the reserved beans and a big pinch of queso fresco. Continue cooking until browned on the bottom, 3–4 minutes more, then transfer to a large platter and tent with foil to keep warm while you finish cooking the rest of the sopes.

5. To serve, drizzle the warm sopes with Salsa Roja. Top each sope with a big pinch of curtido, garnish with cilantro sprigs, if using, and serve warm.

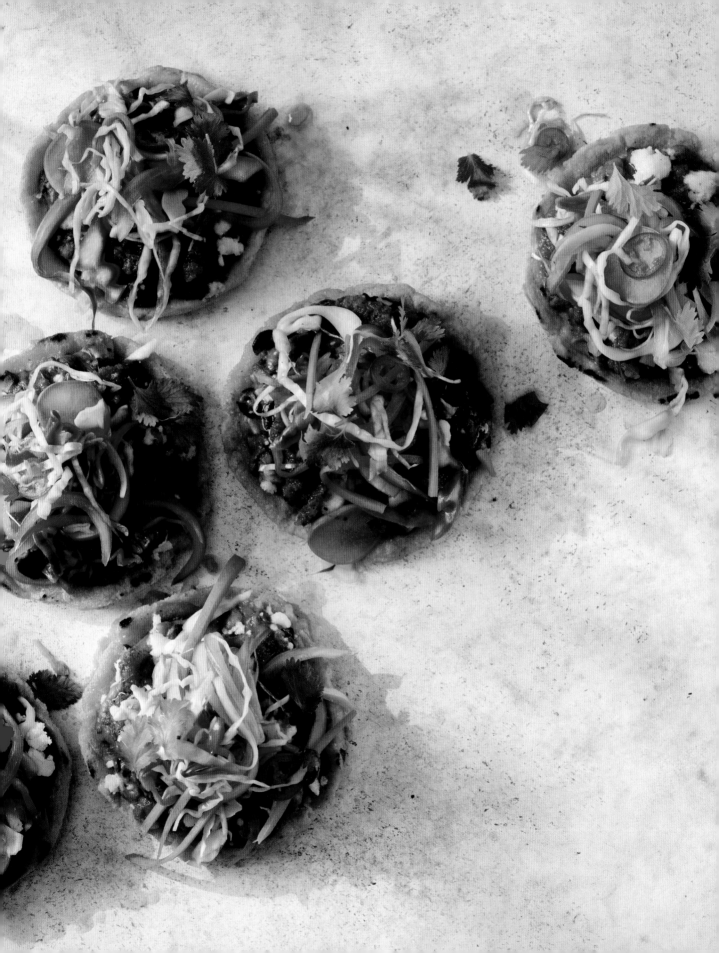

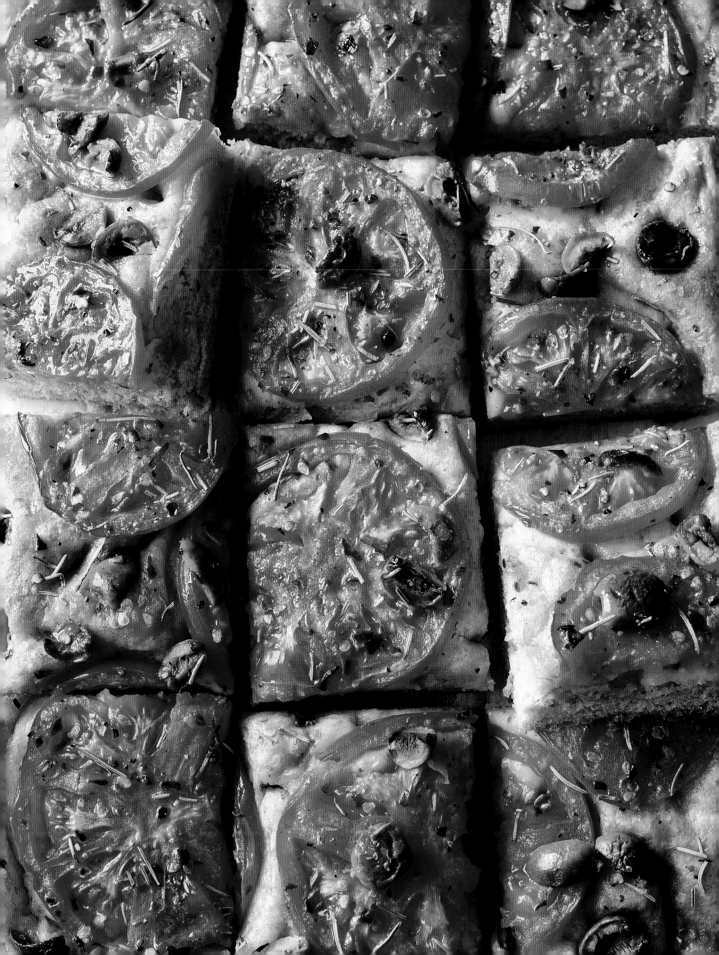

Focaccia
with Beefsteak Tomatoes and Olives

Makes one 13- by 9-inch sheet	Total Time: 1 hr., plus 6 hr. fermentation

FOR THE FOCACCIA

1¼ tsp. instant yeast
(not active dry)

2½ cups (325 g)
all-purpose flour

1 cup (123 g) whole wheat flour

½ cup (80 g) semolina

¼ cup plus 1 Tbsp. extra-virgin
olive oil, divided

1½ tsp. fine sea salt

FOR THE TOPPINGS

2 medium beefsteak tomatoes
(about 1 lb.), thinly sliced

⅓ cup pitted green olives

1 tsp. dried rosemary

1 tsp. dried oregano

1 tsp. dried thyme

1 Tbsp. extra-virgin olive oil

Flaky sea salt

Freshly ground black pepper

Crushed red chile
flakes (optional)

Marie-Pierre is an avid home bread-baker and Kat baked professionally for many years, so we took the bread recipes in this book very seriously. This one uses an extremely versatile dough that lends itself to meal prep and experimentation. A slow, cold fermentation allows its gluten structure to develop gradually, resulting in an irregular and airy open crumb and complex yeasty flavors. We suggest mixing a double batch of the dough ahead of time and storing the extra in the fridge or freezer for up to a month to use as a base for last-minute pizzas, calzones, or grilled flatbreads.

Environmental differences and variations in ingredients can have an impact on fermentation. Remember that the rising times listed in any yeasted recipes are always approximations. For the best results, keep an eye on the visual and tactile cues described throughout.

1. **Make the focaccia:** In the bowl of a stand mixer fitted with a dough hook, mix 1½ cups of cool water and the yeast. Add the flours and semolina and mix on low speed until a shaggy dough forms, about 1 minute. Turn the mixer off, pour 1 Tbsp. of the oil and the salt over the dough, and set aside to rest for 15 minutes.

2. Turn the mixer to second speed and continue mixing until the salt and oil are incorporated and the dough is very smooth, 3–4 minutes more. Cover the bowl with a lid or plastic wrap and set in a warm place until the dough is soft and slightly airy, about 1 hour (it will not yet be doubled in size). Keep an eye on it. If the room is warm, this may happen more quickly.

—continued—

3. Uncover the bowl, then, without taking the dough out of the bowl, gently stretch the dough up and over itself a few times, essentially folding it. Re-cover the bowl and transfer to the fridge for at least 4 and up to 24 hours (or freeze for up to 30 days).

4. When you're ready to bake the focaccia, pour the remaining ¼ cup of olive oil into a 13- by 9-inch rimmed baking sheet and, using clean hands, smear it around to coat the bottom and sides of the pan. Turn the cold dough onto the pan and press down to deflate it. Flip the dough over so that it is oiled on both sides, then use your hands to flatten it to an even layer (the dough won't yet reach all the way to the edges of the pan). Cover loosely with plastic wrap, then set aside in a warm place until very soft and gassy, 40–50 minutes.

5. Meanwhile, make the toppings: Position a rack in the center of the oven and preheat it to 425°F. In a medium bowl, toss the tomato slices, olives, rosemary, oregano, thyme, and oil to combine. Season lightly with salt and black pepper and set aside.

6. Uncover the focaccia and gently stretch the dough to fill the baking sheet. Poke the dough all over with your fingers to dimple and spread it to an even thickness without deflating. Arrange and gently press the tomato slices and olives into the dough and drizzle any remaining juices over the surface. Sprinkle with the chile flakes, if using, then set aside until the dough puffs up around the toppings, 20–30 minutes.

7. Bake until the focaccia is light golden brown at the edges and crisped and golden on the bottom, 30–35 minutes. Cool slightly, then cut into strips and serve warm or at room temperature.

Mushroom "Carbonara"
with Broccoli Rabe and Parmesan

Serves 4–6	Total Time: 35 min.

4 large eggs

1 Tbsp. miso

½ oz. finely grated Parmesan cheese, plus more for serving

1 Tbsp. fresh lemon juice, plus lemon wedges for serving

½ tsp. freshly ground black pepper

Kosher salt

1 Tbsp. extra-virgin olive oil

1 medium shallot, thinly sliced

8 oz. mixed mushrooms, cleaned, trimmed, and sliced or torn into bite-sized pieces

3 garlic cloves, thinly sliced

1 lb. whole wheat spaghetti

8 oz. broccoli rabe (rapini), trimmed, torn into bite-sized pieces, thick stalks coarsely chopped

Crushed red chile flakes (optional)

In our sleep-healthy ode to the beloved Roman pasta dish, meaty mushrooms stand in for the traditional cured pork. A dollop of miso and a handful of grated Parm lend the sauce its obligatory savory richness. Ordinary button or cremini mushrooms work nicely, but if your market stocks a wider variety, oyster, hen-of-the-woods, and shiitake are particularly lovely in this dish. If using shiitake, remove the tough stems before using the tender caps. (Discard the stems, or save for infusing flavor into soups and stocks.)

1. In a medium bowl, whisk together the eggs, miso, Parmesan, lemon juice, and black pepper and set aside. Bring a large pot of salted water to a boil.

2. Meanwhile, cook the mushrooms: In a large skillet, heat the oil over medium heat until it begins to shimmer. Add the shallot and cook, stirring occasionally, until softened and very lightly browned, 3–4 minutes. Add the mushrooms and garlic and cook, stirring occasionally, until tender and browned, 6–8 minutes more. (If the mushrooms start to seem dry and stick to the skillet before they have softened, stir in ¼ cup of water, scraping the browned bits off the bottom of the skillet, and continue cooking until the mushrooms are tender.) Remove from heat and set aside.

3. Add the pasta to the boiling water and cook, stirring frequently, until just barely softened, about 4 minutes. Ladle out 1½ cups of the pasta-cooking water, then stir in the broccoli rabe and cook until the spaghetti is al dente and the greens are tender-crisp and still bright green, 4–6 minutes more.

—continued—

4. Strain, discarding the cooking liquid, then return the pasta and broccoli rabe to the pot. Stir the reserved pasta-cooking water into the egg mixture, then add that and the reserved mushroom mixture to the pot. Stir immediately to combine—the heat from the pasta will begin to thicken the egg to a light and creamy sauce, but if necessary, return to low heat and cook, stirring and scraping the bottom of the pot continuously, until the sauce thickens, 2–3 minutes. Remove from heat and divide among wide pasta bowls. Finish with a squeeze of lemon juice, some more Parmesan, and a pinch of crushed red chile flakes, if using, and serve warm.

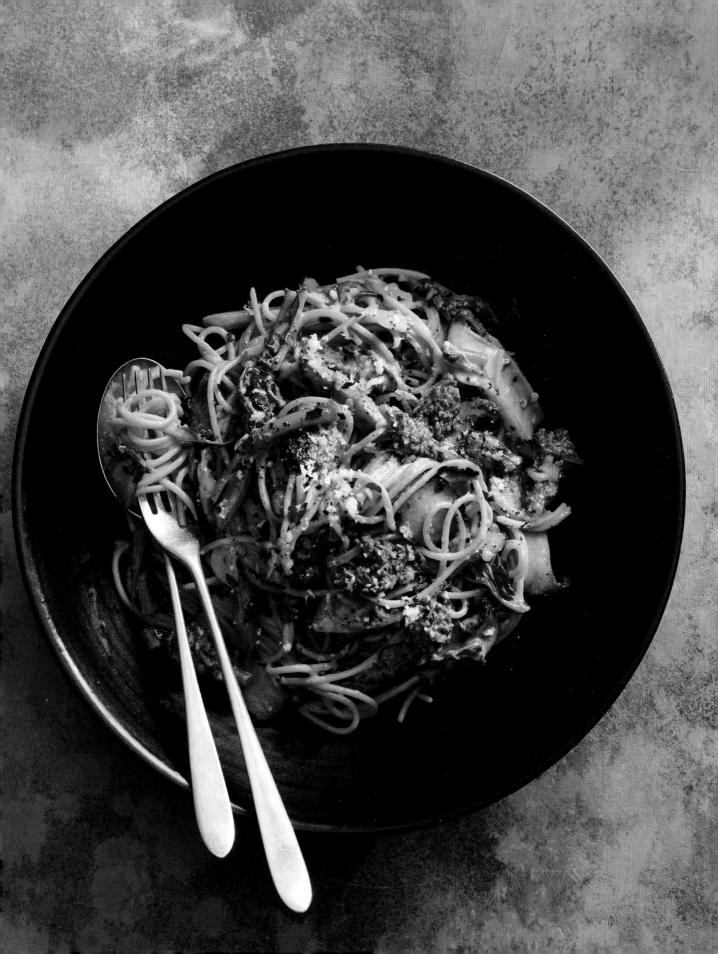

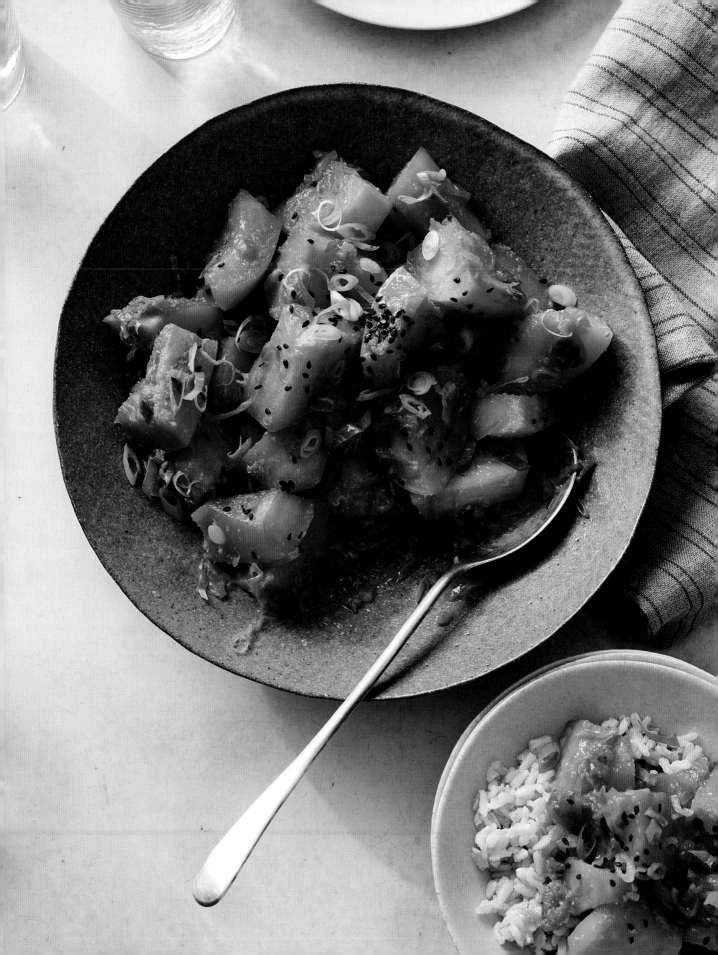

Soy-Braised Butternut Squash
with Miso Butter and Black Sesame

Serves 2–4	Total Time: 30 min.

1 Tbsp. Miso Butter (page 123) (or substitute 2 tsp. salted butter plus 1 tsp. sesame oil)

1 Tbsp. finely grated fresh ginger

4 medium scallions, trimmed and thinly sliced (⅓ cup), plus more for sprinkling

⅓ cup low-sodium chicken or mushroom stock

2 Tbsp. low-sodium soy sauce

2 Tbsp. honey

Pinch of crushed red chile flakes (optional)

One 1¼-lb. butternut squash, peeled, seeded, and cut into 1½-in. pieces

1 tsp. black sesame seeds

Umami-rich miso and soy sauce lend sweet and starchy winter squash an unexpected savory depth in this simple, Asian-inspired braise. We like to pair this with classic roast turkey or chicken; once the bird is out of the oven and resting, get the squash started. It comes together in 30 minutes and with very little mess.

1. In a medium skillet or wide pot, heat the Miso Butter over medium heat until it begins to sizzle. Add the ginger and scallions and cook, stirring frequently, until the scallions are softened and the ginger is very fragrant, 1–2 minutes. Stir in the stock, soy sauce, honey, and chile flakes, if using, and bring to a simmer, then add the squash and cook, stirring occasionally, until slightly softened, about 8 minutes. Turn the heat to low, cover, and continue cooking until the squash is tender when poked with a fork, 8-10 minutes more.

2. Remove from heat, stir gently, then transfer to a wide bowl. Sprinkle with black sesame seeds and scallions, and serve.

Chickpea Gemelli
with Butternut Squash, Walnuts, and Parmesan

Serves 3–4

Total Time: 1 hr.

Kosher salt

8 oz. dried chickpea
gemelli or other pasta

1 Tbsp. extra-virgin olive oil

8 fresh sage leaves

One 1-lb butternut squash,
seeded, peeled, and cut in
½-in. cubes (about 2 cups)

1 small yellow onion,
coarsely chopped

4 garlic cloves, thinly sliced

½ cup dry white wine

1 cup chicken or
mushroom stock

⅓ cup coarsely grated
Parmesan cheese

2 Tbsp. coarsely chopped
walnuts (optional)

Smoked paprika or freshly
ground black pepper

Chickpea pasta is a delicious, high-protein, high-fiber, and gluten-free alternative to wheat-based macaroni. We find that its hearty texture works well in this cozy autumn dish, but if you can't track it down, whole wheat versions work great here, too—just adjust the pasta cooking time according to the package instructions. Serve this dish with a green salad on the side to make it a full meal.

1. Bring a large pot of salted water to a boil, then add the pasta and cook, stirring occasionally, for 5 minutes; it will still be quite al dente at this point. Reserve 1 cup of the cooking liquid, then drain the pasta and set aside.

2. Return the pot to medium-high heat and add the oil. When the oil begins to shimmer, add the sage leaves and cook, stirring frequently, until fragrant and crispy, 2–4 minutes. Remove the leaves from the pot and set aside. To the same pot, add the squash, onion, and garlic, lower the heat to medium, and cook, stirring frequently, until the squash is just tender when poked with a fork, 8–10 minutes. Stir in the wine, using a wooden spoon to scrape up any browned bits from the bottom of the pot; cook until the alcohol has boiled off, 4–5 minutes, then add the stock and the reserved pasta water. Increase the heat to medium-high, bring to a boil, and continue cooking until the squash is very soft, about 10 minutes more.

3. Remove from heat and blend the vegetable mixture with an immersion blender until smooth. (Alternatively, transfer the mixture to a jug blender, blend until smooth, then return the purée to the pot.) Stir in the pasta, return to medium heat, and bring to a boil. Cook, stirring gently, until the pasta is just tender and the sauce is slightly thickened, 2–3 minutes more. Remove from heat and stir in half of the Parmesan. Ladle the pasta into wide bowls, top with the remaining Parmesan, walnuts, if using, and the reserved sage leaves. Sprinkle with smoked paprika or black pepper and serve hot.

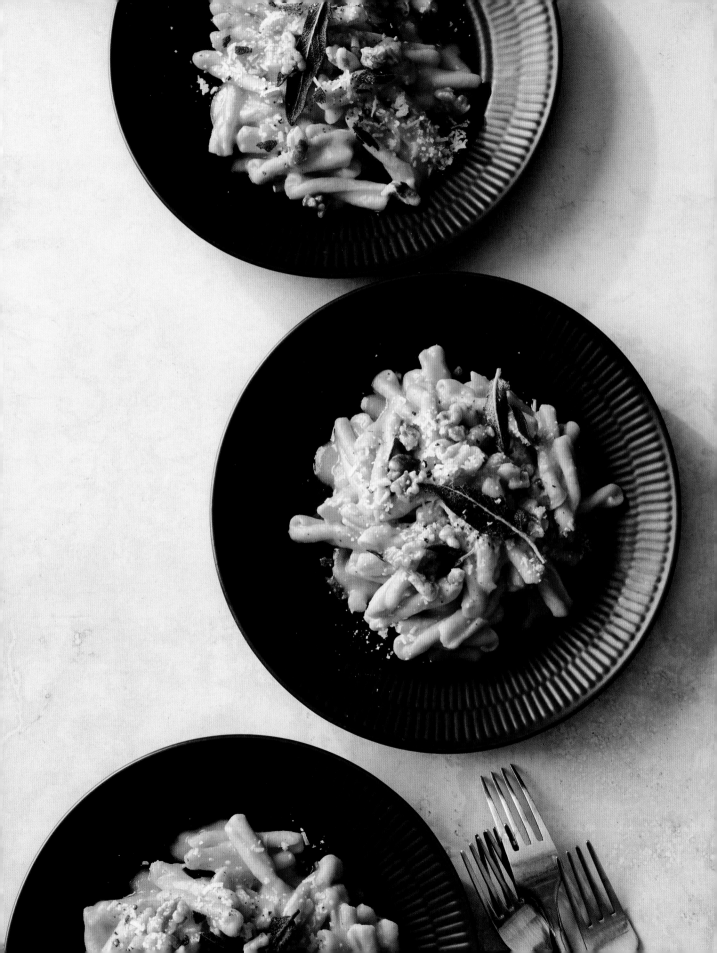

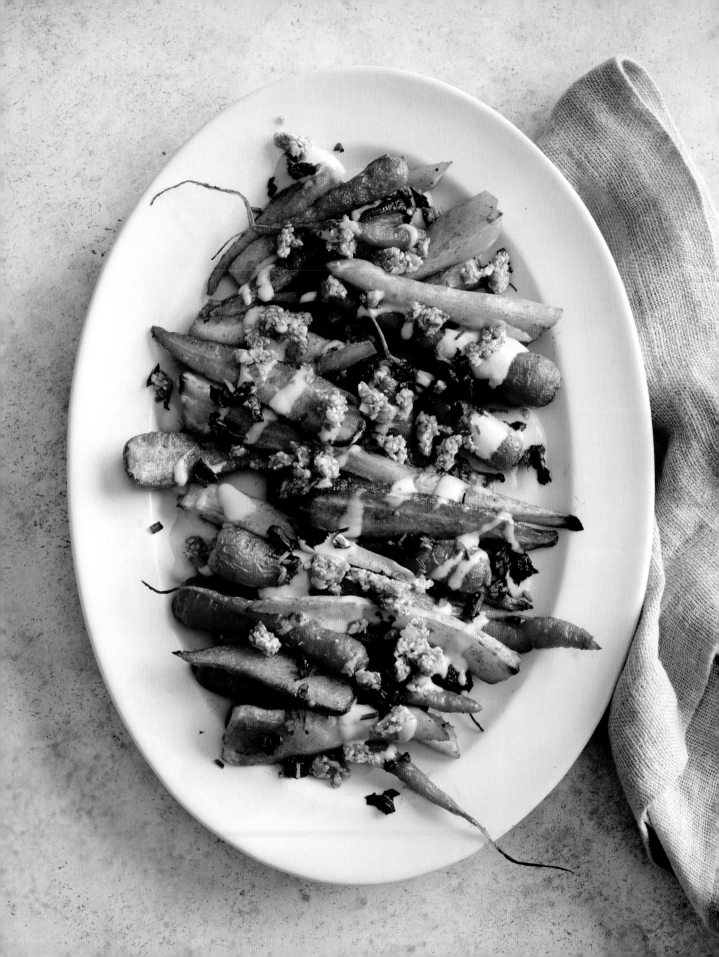

Spiced Carrots and Parsnips
with Tahini-Lemon Sauce

Serves 4

Total Time: 50 min.

1 lb. parsnips, peeled

1½ lb. carrots, peeled

1 Tbsp. extra-virgin olive oil

½ tsp. ground cinnamon

½ tsp. ground coriander

½ tsp. ground cumin

½ tsp. kosher salt,
plus more to taste

¼ cup tahini

2 Tbsp. fresh lemon juice

1 large garlic clove, finely grated

¼ cup Sesame-Cashew
Crunch (page 104)

1 tsp. Herbs Salées (page
117) (or substitute finely
chopped fresh parsley)

Carrots and parsnips keep so well in a plastic bag in the fridge that they're effectively a pantry staple. This recipe is a breeze to throw together and a great way to get fresh veggies on the table when you haven't had an opportunity to get to the market in a while. If you don't have a batch of Sesame-Cashew Crunch prepared, lightly toasted slivered almonds work nicely in this dish, too.

1. Preheat the oven to 400°F.

2. Cut any thick parsnips or carrots lengthwise so the roots are generally alike in thickness. Place the root vegetables on a large rimmed baking sheet and rub them all over with the olive oil. Sprinkle with the cinnamon, coriander, cumin, and salt, then bake, stirring occasionally, until the carrots and parsnips are tender when poked with a fork and lightly browned, 30–40 minutes.

3. Meanwhile, make the tahini sauce: In a small bowl, whisk together the tahini, lemon juice, and garlic (the sauce will thicken and seize up at first; don't worry, it will loosen up as you mix). Stir in 2–3 tablespoons of cool water until the sauce thins to a pourable consistency. Season to taste with salt.

4. Transfer the carrots and parsnips to a platter, drizzle with the tahini sauce, sprinkle with Sesame-Cashew Crunch and Herbes Salées, and serve warm.

Cold Marinated Tofu
with Sesame and Scallions

Serves 4 | Total Time: 10 min.

¼ cup soy sauce

1 Tbsp. mirin

1 Tbsp. sesame oil

1½ tsp. rice vinegar

3 scallions, thinly sliced, plus more for garnish (optional)

2 tsp. sesame seeds

One 12-oz. block silken or soft tofu, drained and cut in ½-in. cubes

½–1 tsp. chile oil (optional)

Inspired by a popular Japanese summertime dish, this quick and protein-rich vegan recipe is perfect for those steamy summer evenings when the last thing you want to do is turn on the stove. Tofu is a great source of protein and sleep-supporting tryptophan. Make this dish a light meal by pairing it with warm brown rice and a side of steamed leafy greens with Creamy Sesame-Ginger Vinaigrette (page 115). If you're sensitive to chiles, omit the chile oil and replace it with some grated fresh ginger.

1. In a small bowl, stir together the soy sauce, mirin, sesame oil, vinegar, scallions, and sesame seeds.

2. Arrange the tofu on a large rimmed plate or a wide, shallow bowl. Pour the dressing over the cubes, drizzle with chile oil and scallions, if using, and serve cold.

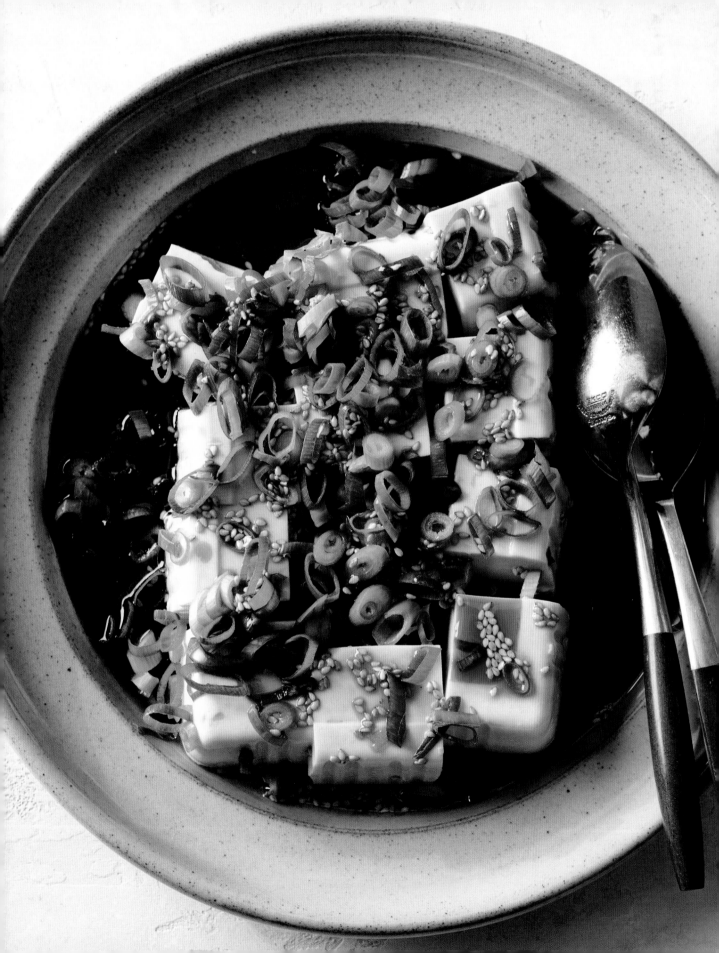

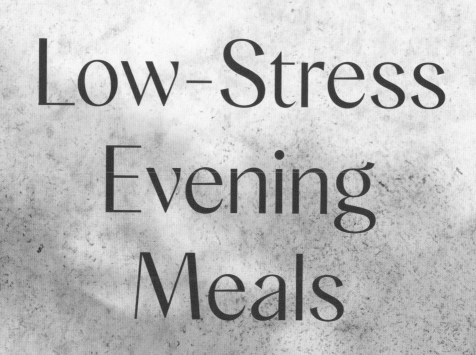

Low-Stress Evening Meals

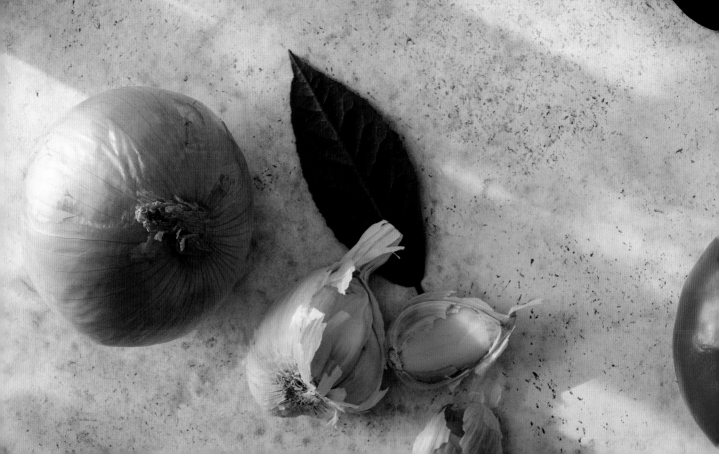

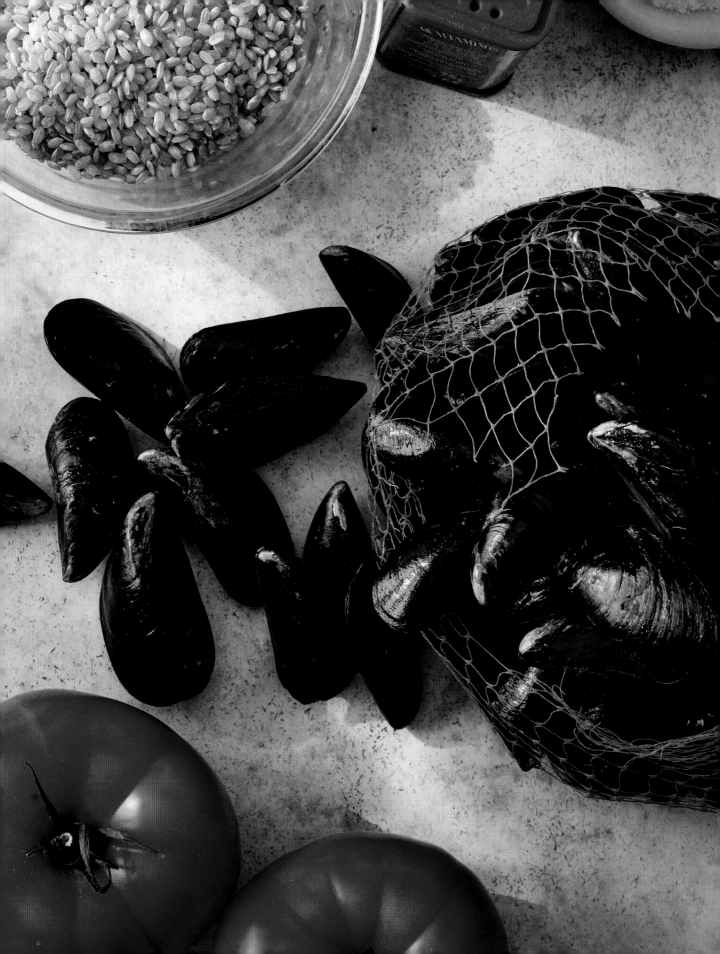

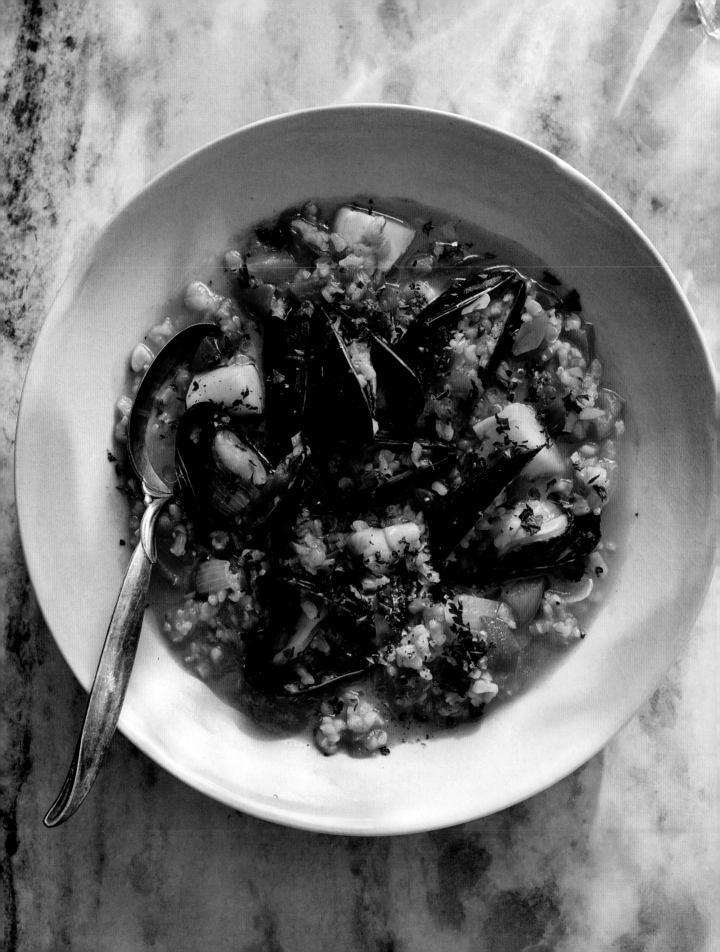

Portuguese-Style Tomato Rice
with Mussels and Scallops

Serves 4

Total Time: 1 hr. 30 min.

2 Tbsp. extra-virgin olive oil

1 medium red bell pepper, stemmed, seeded, and coarsely chopped

1 medium yellow onion, coarsely chopped

3 garlic cloves, coarsely chopped

2 tsp. smoked paprika (optional)

1 bay leaf

Kosher salt and freshly ground black pepper

3 large beefsteak tomatoes (about 1½ lb.), coarsely chopped, juices reserved

1¼ cups short-grain brown rice

½ cup dry white wine

3 cups clam broth or low-sodium fish stock (or substitute water)

1 lb. mussels, cleaned

12 oz. whole bay scallops or sea scallops, cut in 1-in. pieces

¼ cup finely chopped fresh parsley

This sleep-supporting nutritional powerhouse of a meal is based on a Portuguese dish traditionally made with octopus, an ingredient that also happens to be loaded with tryptophan and lean protein. If your local fishmonger has them, feel free to swap out all or some of the shellfish in this recipe for an equal portion of cooked octopus tentacles. In a pinch, cooked tinned octopus, which is widely available in Latin American and Mediterranean markets, works nicely, too. If tomatoes, alliums, or peppers cause you to experience acid reflux, you're probably better off skipping this one, or at least avoiding it and other aggravating foods after lunchtime.

1. In a wide pot, heat the oil over medium heat until it begins to shimmer. Add the bell pepper, onion, and garlic and cook, stirring frequently, until softened and very fragrant, 5–7 minutes. Stir in the paprika, if using, add the bay leaf, and season lightly with salt and black pepper, then add the tomatoes and cook, stirring occasionally, until concentrated and jammy, about 15 minutes.

2. Stir in the rice, then add the wine and cook until the alcohol boils off, 1–2 minutes. Stir in the clam broth and 1 cup of water, increase the heat to high, bring the liquid up to a full boil, then lower the heat to medium-low and simmer, stirring occasionally, until the rice is tender, 40–45 minutes.

3. Stir the pot well, then add the mussels and scallops, cover, and cook just until the mussels have opened and the scallops are barely cooked, about 5 minutes. Season to taste with additional salt and black pepper, then divide into wide soup bowls, top with parsley, and serve hot.

Provençal Stuffed Tomatoes

Serves 4

Total Time: 1 hr. 20 min.

4 medium beefsteak
or large vine-ripened
tomatoes (about 2 lb.)

Kosher salt and freshly
ground black pepper

3 Tbsp. extra-virgin
olive oil, divided

Two 3-oz. Italian-style chicken
sausages, casings removed

1 small yellow onion,
finely chopped

3 garlic cloves, finely grated

2 tsp. herbes de Provence

1½ cups cooked brown rice

⅓ cup coarsely chopped
fresh parsley

3 Tbsp. freshly grated
Parmesan cheese

In 2020, a study on tomatoes, a known dietary source of melatonin, showed that postmenopausal women who ate beefsteak tomatoes every day for eight weeks slept better and had increased melatonin production compared to a control group that had been given no tomatoes.

For this attractive dish, select large tomatoes that are ripe and unblemished but still firm; overly juicy ones tend to turn to mush as they bake. Feel free to assemble the tomatoes ahead of time—just wrap them tightly in plastic and refrigerate for up to 3 days before you plan to serve. If baking straight from the fridge, allow for an additional 10–15 minutes in the oven.

1. Cut ½ inch off the stem end of the tomatoes, reserving the tops. Use a spoon to carefully scoop out their insides without breaking the outer walls. Coarsely chop the pulp and transfer it to a bowl, along with any juices. Sprinkle the insides of the tomatoes lightly with salt and black pepper.

2. Drizzle 1 tablespoon of the olive oil into a large baking dish. Place the tomatoes cut-side up in the dish and rub them all over with the oil. Rub their lids with some of the oil as well, then set aside.

3. Preheat the oven to 275°F. In a medium cast-iron skillet or other heavy skillet, heat the remaining oil over medium heat until it begins to shimmer. Add the sausage and cook, stirring and breaking up the meat occasionally, until cooked through and beginning to brown, 3–4 minutes. Add the onion and continue cooking until translucent, about 5 minutes more. Stir in the garlic and herbes de Provence and cook until fragrant, about 1 minute. Stir in the reserved tomato pulp and any accumulated juices, scraping the bottom of the skillet with a wooden spoon. Continue cooking until the mixture has the consistency of a chunky sauce, 12–15 minutes.

4. Transfer the sausage-and-tomato mixture to a large, heatproof bowl. Stir in the rice, parsley, and Parmesan, season to taste with more salt and black pepper, then scoop into the reserved tomatoes. (Fill them, but do not pack the filling tightly.) Place the tomatoes' lids back on, then transfer the dish, uncovered, to the oven and bake until the filling is very hot and the tomatoes are tender when poked with a fork, 25–30 minutes. Serve hot or at room temperature.

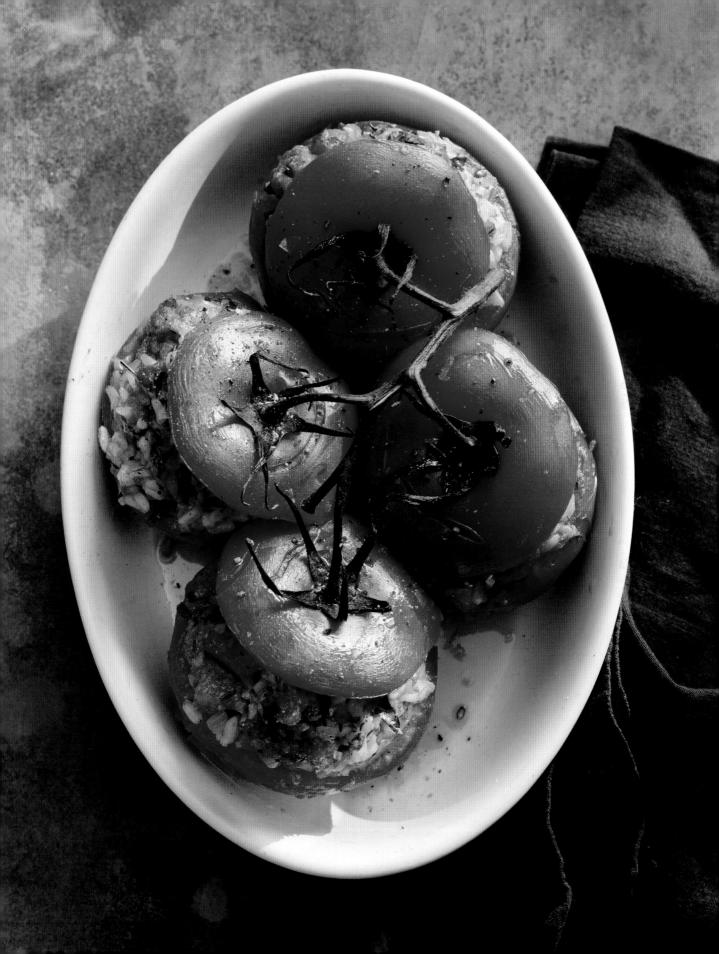

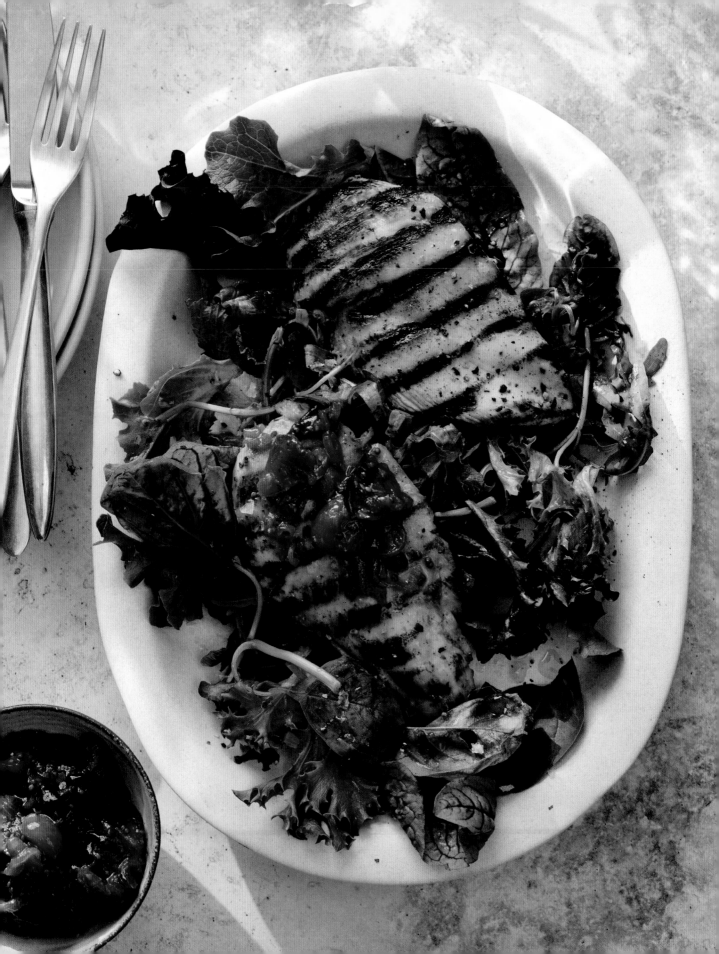

Grilled Chicken Cutlets
with Midsummer Mostarda

| Serves 2 | Total Time: 1 hr. 15 min. |

FOR THE MARINADE

2 Tbsp. red wine vinegar
or apple cider vinegar

2 garlic cloves, finely grated

2 tsp. dried oregano

1½ tsp. fish sauce

Freshly ground black pepper

Pinch of crushed red
chile flakes (optional)

¼ cup extra-virgin olive oil

½ lb. boneless, skinless
chicken breast, cut
crosswise into approximately
½-in.-thick cutlets

FOR THE MOSTARDA

½ tsp. extra-virgin olive oil

½ small shallot, thinly sliced

⅓ cup Midsummer
Compote (page 98)

1½ tsp. grainy mustard

1½ tsp. honey

Kosher salt

FOR SERVING

4 cups arugula or
mixed baby greens

Boneless, skinless chicken breast is a blank canvas. If you're anti-white meat, the easy and adaptable marinade in this recipe may inspire you to give the lean and tryptophan-rich protein another chance. Sensitive to spice? Omit the chile flakes. Out of vinegar? Use lemon or lime juice instead. Afraid of fish sauce? Well, don't be. But if you still are, replace it with half a teaspoon of salt. No grill? No sweat—just throw these babies on a grill pan or under the broiler. One hour is all you need to impart chicken breast with plenty of flavor, but if you prefer to get a head start, you can let it sit in the fridge for up to eight. Still not convinced? Well, that's okay: This whole recipe works great with center-cut boneless pork chops, too!

Mostarda is a mustard-flavored sweet-and-savory Italian condiment often served with cheeses and roasted meats. We make our summery version by dressing up the gingery Midsummer Compote from the Pantry chapter. For a more classic version, start with the Winter Compote (page 100) or even a jar of store-bought fig jam instead.

1. **Make the marinade:** In a wide bowl, combine the vinegar, garlic, oregano, fish sauce, black pepper, and chile flakes, if using. Whisk in the olive oil, then add the chicken cutlets, turning once or twice to thoroughly coat. Cover with plastic wrap, transfer to the fridge, and marinate for at least 1 and up to 8 hours.

2. **Make the mostarda:** In a small pot, heat the oil over medium heat until it begins to shimmer. Add the shallot and cook, stirring frequently, until softened and just beginning to brown, 2–3 minutes. Stir in the compote, bring to a simmer, lower the heat to medium-low, and cook until the shallots are very soft, 2–4 minutes. Stir in

—continued—

the mustard and honey and continue cooking until the juices are thickened, 3–5 minutes more. Remove from heat, season to taste with salt, and set aside.

3. Light a grill to cook over medium-high heat or preheat a grill pan over high heat. When the grill is hot, add the chicken and grill, flipping once, until cooked through, 5–7 minutes.

4. Arrange the arugula or baby greens on a serving platter, then place the chicken on top. Serve warm, with mostarda on the side.

Lamb Stew
with Bulgur, Almonds, Dried Fruit, and Fresh Herbs

Serves 6	Total Time: 1 hr. 45 min.

1¾ lb. boneless lamb stew meat, excess fat trimmed, cut into 1-in. cubes

Kosher salt and freshly ground black pepper

2 Tbsp. extra-virgin olive oil

5 medium shallots, peeled and halved lengthwise

8 garlic cloves, thinly sliced

3 Tbsp. finely grated fresh ginger

1 bay leaf

1½ tsp. ground cinnamon

1½ tsp. ground cumin

¾ tsp. ground turmeric

Pinch of saffron, soaked in 1 Tbsp. warm water (optional)

1 large beefsteak tomato, cored and coarsely chopped

6 dried apricots, halved

6 pitted prunes, coarsely chopped

—ingredients continue—

While it would be traditional to serve this Moroccan-style braise over couscous, we drew inspiration from Paris-based food writer David Lebovitz, who serves his version over equally quick-cooking—and far more nutrient-rich—bulgur. Lamb is exceptionally high in tryptophan and is also an excellent source of several essential nutrients, including zinc and vitamin B_6, two of the four essential nutrients involved in the body's production of serotonin and melatonin.

1. Season the lamb lightly with salt and black pepper. In a large heavy pot, heat the oil over medium-high heat until it begins to shimmer. Add the lamb and cook, stirring occasionally, until browned all over, 8–10 minutes. Transfer the meat to a heatproof bowl and set aside.

2. Return the pot to medium-high heat, then add the shallots, cut-side down, and cook until lightly browned on one side, 3–4 minutes. Stir in the garlic and ginger and cook until fragrant, about 30 seconds. Add the bay leaf, cinnamon, cumin, turmeric, and saffron water, if using, then stir in the tomatoes and 1 cup of water. Bring to a boil, then return the lamb to the pot. Lower the heat to simmer, cover, and cook for 20 minutes.

3. Uncover, sprinkle the apricots and prunes over the stew, cover once again, and continue cooking until the meat is very tender, 30–40 minutes more.

—continued—

FOR SERVING

6 cups cooked bulgur (see sidebar for cooking instructions)

⅓ cup sliced almonds, lightly toasted

Coarsely chopped fresh herbs, such as mint, cilantro, parsley, or scallion, for garnish

Aleppo pepper or crushed red chile flakes (optional)

¼ cup plain yogurt (optional)

Lemon wedges

Bulgur—the coarsely chopped whole wheat most commonly used in tabbouleh, is a quick-cooking whole-grain alternative to couscous. To prepare, add **2 cups of medium-ground bulgur** to a large pot. Add 3 cups of cool water, set over medium-high heat, and bring to a simmer. Cover, turn down the heat to low, and cook until the liquid is absorbed, 12–14 minutes. Remove from the heat and set aside, covered, for 5 minutes. Uncover, sprinkle with **1 tablespoon of Herbes Salées (page 117)** or **a handful of fresh herbs** and ½ **teaspoon of fine sea salt,** and fluff with a fork to combine.

4. Remove from heat and season to taste with additional salt and black pepper. Ladle over wide bowls of bulgur and top with almonds, herbs, and a sprinkling of Aleppo pepper and a dollop of yogurt, if using. Serve with lemon wedges, for squeezing.

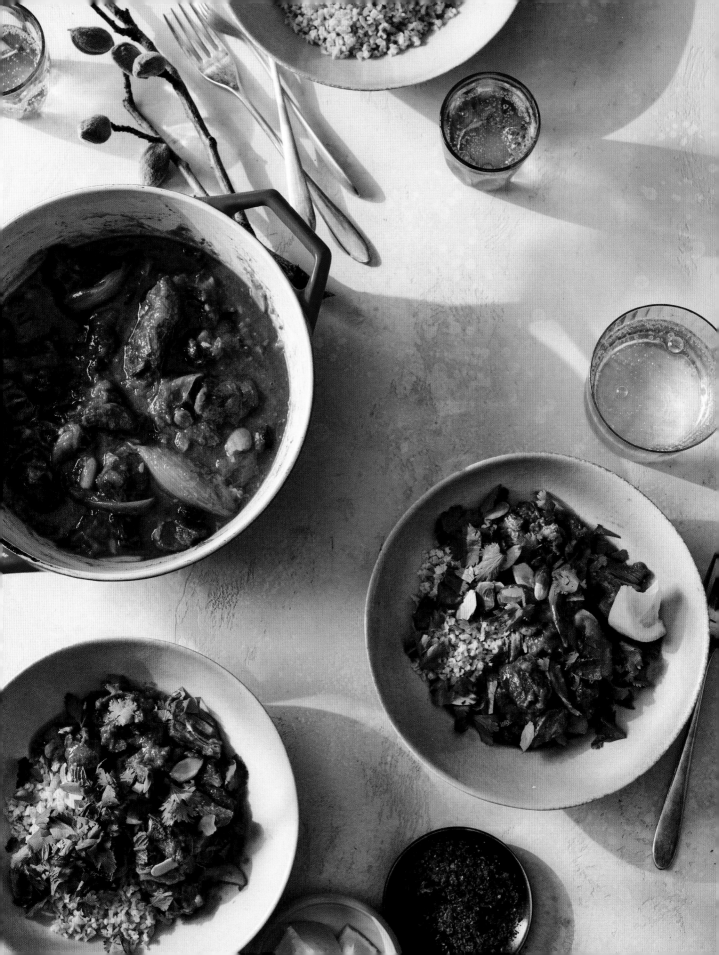

Green Spring Gumbo
with Chicken Andouille

Serves 4–6	Total Time: 1 hr. 30 min.

2 Tbsp. olive oil

Three 2½-oz. chicken andouille sausages, sliced ½ in. thick

2 Tbsp. whole wheat flour

2 medium yellow onions, finely chopped

2 bunches scallions, trimmed and thinly sliced

2 celery stalks, finely chopped

1 green bell pepper, cored, seeded, and finely chopped

2 bay leaves

Kosher salt and freshly ground black pepper

2 tsp. garlic powder

2 tsp. dried thyme

1 tsp. dried oregano

½–1 tsp. cayenne pepper (optional)

This nutrient-rich, vegetable-forward stew is a riff on a style of Creole gumbo traditionally made vegetarian for Lent. It's also a great way to use up a crisper drawer full of greens and fresh herbs. We like to add a little bit of andouille-style chicken sausage for a hit of protein and tryptophan, but if you prefer a pescatarian option, leave out the sausage, replace the chicken stock with mushroom or vegetable broth, and top the finished dish with a few shrimp or even steamed crab or lobster claws. For a vegan option, replace the sausage with tempeh or a spicy or smoked plant-based sausage. Served with brown rice, any of these variations makes a well-balanced and sleep-supporting meal. Leftovers keep well in the freezer.

1. In a large heavy pot, heat the oil over medium heat until it begins to shimmer. Add the sausage and cook, stirring occasionally, until browned, 6–8 minutes. Use a slotted spoon to transfer the sausage to a heatproof bowl and reserve. Lower the heat to medium-low, then stir the flour into the oil that remains in the pot and cook, stirring frequently, just until the mixture, or roux, smells toasty, about 5 minutes. Add the onions, scallions, celery, bell pepper, and bay leaves, season lightly with salt and black pepper, and cook, stirring and scraping the bottom of the pot frequently, until the onions are translucent, 12–14 minutes.

1¼ lb. mixed greens and fresh herbs, such as spinach, arugula, collards, kale, Swiss chard, broccoli rabe, parsley, and cilantro, chopped

4 cups chicken stock

3 cups cooked brown rice

Lemon wedges, for serving

2. Stir in the garlic powder, thyme, oregano, and cayenne, if using, then add the greens a little at a time, allowing them to wilt before adding more, until they all fit in the pot. Stir in the chicken stock. Increase the heat to medium-high, bring the liquid to a full boil, and then decrease the heat to low, cover, and simmer, stirring occasionally, until the broth has thickened and the greens are almost meltingly tender and have turned from bright green to a muted olive color, 30–45 minutes (if you're using hardier greens like collards, they will take a bit longer to cook, while softer varieties like baby spinach will cook quickly).

3. Stir in the reserved sausage, cover, and continue cooking for 15 minutes more. Adjust the seasoning with more salt and black pepper, then ladle into soup bowls. Top each bowl with a scoop of rice and a lemon wedge and serve hot.

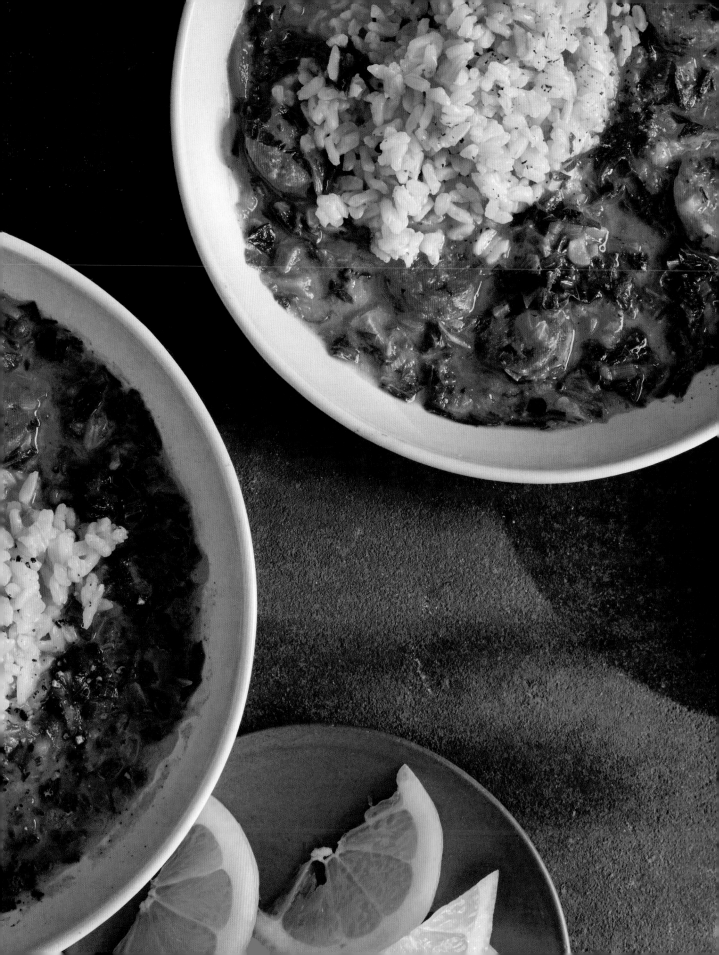

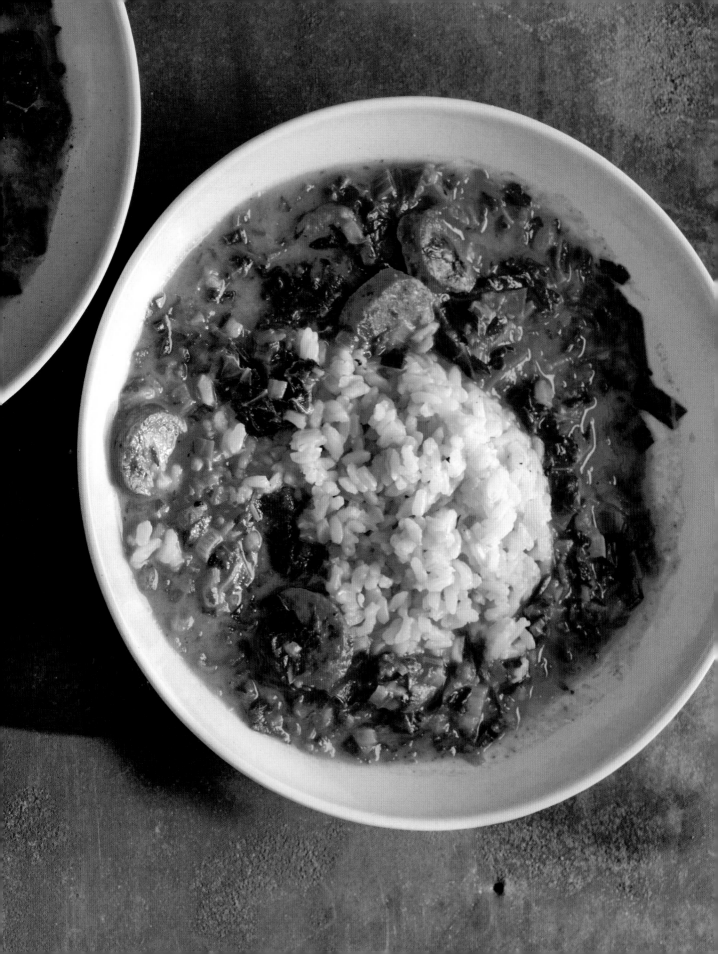

Whole Grain Chicken Porridge
with Scallions and Sesame-Cashew Crunch

Serves 6 | Total Time: 1 hr. 20 min.

One 1-lb. chicken leg quarter, skin removed

¾ cup brown rice

½ cup pearl barley

½ cup rolled (old-fashioned) oats

⅓ cup finely chopped fresh ginger

1 Tbsp. plus 1 tsp. Chinese five-spice powder

2 small onions, coarsely chopped

2 cups sliced mushrooms

1 cup coarsely chopped celery

2 medium carrots, peeled and coarsely chopped

6 garlic cloves

1 Tbsp. soy sauce

Kosher salt

1 cup thinly sliced scallions

¾ cup Sesame-Cashew Crunch (page 104) or salted, crushed peanuts

Crushed red chile flakes (optional)

1 Tbsp. sesame oil

Savory rice porridges are enjoyed as a simple homestyle meal throughout much of Asia, where they may be flavored with poultry, meat, or seafood, and topped with any assortment of fresh, spicy, or crunchy toppings. We made our own version of this soothing and economical comfort food using a mix of tryptophan- and fiber-rich whole grains and dark-meat chicken. One good-sized leg quarter (drumstick plus thigh) goes a long way; feel free to swap in an equivalent weight of skinless chicken thighs, drumsticks, or even one big turkey drum. Resist the urge to cut fat and calories by using chicken breast for this one—the small amount of fat in the dark meat gets distributed among many servings.

This style of porridge is often eaten in the morning, so if you have a slow cooker, you may want to break it out to cook this one overnight—or set it up in the morning for a made-ahead dinner at the end of the day.

1. In a Dutch oven or large heavy pot, combine the chicken, brown rice, barley, oats, ginger, and five-spice powder. Add 7 cups of cold water, set over medium-high heat, bring to a boil, then add the onions, mushrooms, celery, carrots, and garlic. Cover the pot, lower the heat to low, and cook, stirring and scraping the bottom occasionally, until the chicken is very tender, about 1 hour.

2. Uncover the pot and use tongs to transfer the chicken leg to a plate. Use two forks to remove and discard the bones, then shred the meat into bite-sized pieces and stir it back into the porridge. Stir in the soy sauce, then season to taste with salt. Remove from heat, then ladle the porridge into 6 soup bowls. Top with sliced scallions, Sesame-Cashew Crunch, and chile flakes, if using. Drizzle each bowl with ½ teaspoon of sesame oil and serve hot.

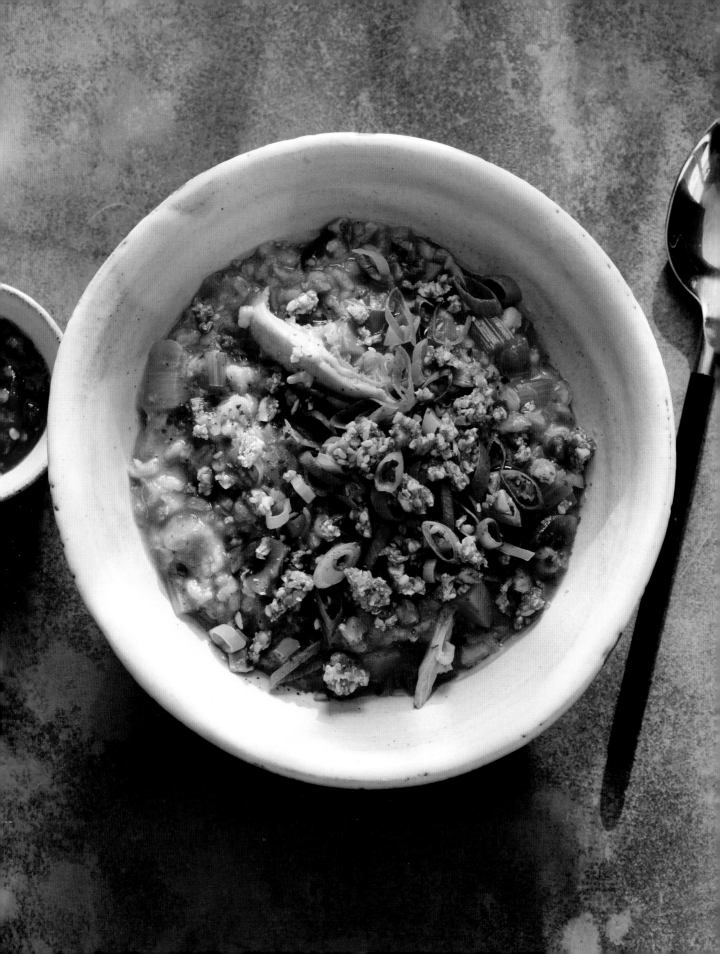

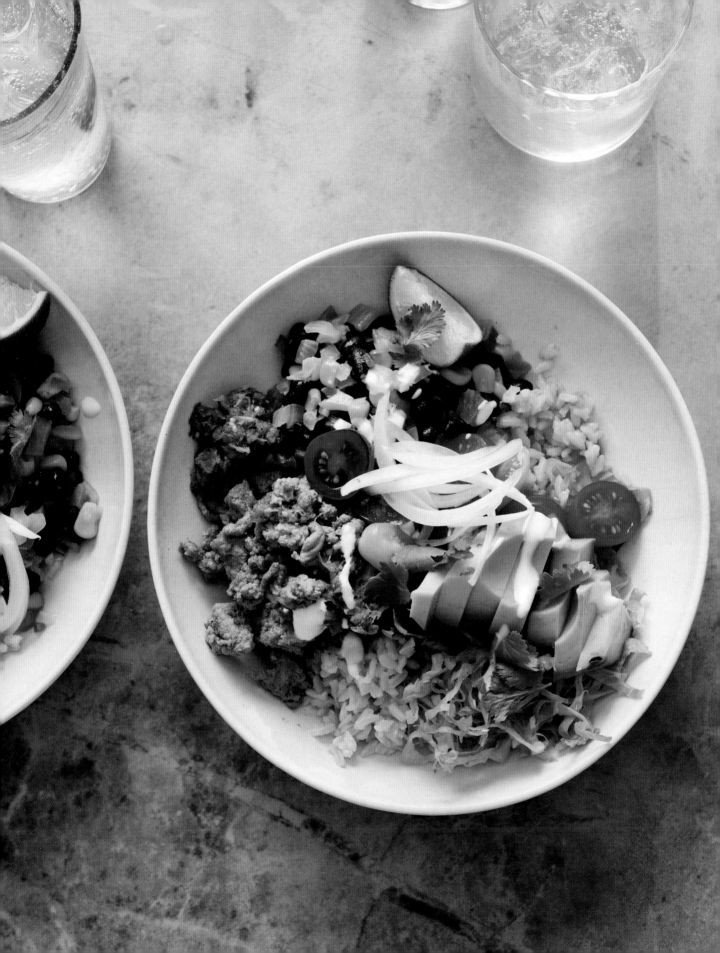

Turkey and Black Bean Burrito Bowl
with Salsa Verde

Serves 4–6	Total Time: 45 min.

1 large white onion, ½ finely chopped, ½ thinly sliced

2 Tbsp. fresh lime juice, divided, plus lime wedges for serving

Kosher salt

¼ cup Greek yogurt

¼ cup buttermilk

2 Tbsp. olive oil, divided

¾ lb. ground turkey

1 tsp. ground cumin

½ tsp. ground coriander

½ tsp. garlic powder

Cayenne pepper (optional)

1¼ cups finely chopped green bell pepper

One 15.5-oz. can black beans, rinsed and drained

¾ cups corn, cut fresh from the cob or thawed, frozen

2 cups steamed brown rice

1 Romaine lettuce heart, thinly sliced

¾ cup halved grape tomatoes

1 cup Salsa Verde (page 126)

1 medium avocado, pitted, peeled, and thinly sliced

Coarsely chopped fresh cilantro (optional)

This recipe may seem like it has an awful lot of ingredients, but consider it a starting point to be adapted based on your preferences and whatever you find in the fridge. Individual ingredients may be swapped out to your and your family's taste and to use up kitchen leftovers: Turkey for chicken, or even thinly sliced steak. Black beans for pinto or cannellini beans. Crema for queso fresco or shredded Monterey Jack. Replace the homemade Salsa Verde for a good-quality bottled version, if you like. If prepping this dish ahead of time, store the components separately and rewarm just before assembling.

1. In a medium bowl, toss the sliced onion with 1 tablespoon of lime juice and a pinch of salt. Set aside. In a small bowl, whisk together the yogurt and buttermilk. Season the crema to taste with salt and refrigerate.

2. In a large heavy skillet, heat 1 tablespoon of oil over medium heat until it begins to shimmer. Add the turkey, cumin, coriander, and garlic powder and cook, stirring frequently, until the meat is evenly browned but still a little bit juicy, 8–10 minutes. Season to taste with cayenne, if using, and kosher salt, remove from heat, and keep warm while you prepare the rest of the ingredients.

3. In a medium pot, heat the remaining oil over medium heat. When the oil begins to shimmer, add the chopped onion and bell pepper and cook, stirring frequently, until softened, 5–7 minutes. Add the beans, corn, and 1 tablespoon of lime juice and cook, stirring frequently, until heated through, about 2 minutes. Season to taste with salt and remove from heat.

4. Spoon the brown rice into soup bowls. Top each serving with the turkey, the bean-and-vegetable-mixture, marinated onions, crema, lettuce, tomatoes, Salsa Verde, and avocado. Garnish with cilantro, if using, and serve warm, with lime.

Lemony Baked Trout

Serves 2

Total Time: 25 min.

2 rainbow trout fillets

1 garlic clove, thinly sliced

1 small lemon, thinly sliced

1 Tbsp. Herbes Salées
(page 117) (or substitute
2 tsp. finely chopped fresh
parsley, cilantro, or scallions
and ½ tsp. kosher salt)

1 Tbsp. extra-virgin olive oil

Freshly ground black pepper

This super-simple weeknight recipe works well with any thin fish fillets, though we're especially fond of rainbow trout. The low-mercury and easy-to-cook species is particularly high in omega-3 fatty acids. Pair it with a chunk of crusty bread for soaking up the lemony juices and a serving of sautéed greens to make it a meal.

1. Position a rack in the center of the oven and preheat it to 400°F.

2. Line a rimmed baking sheet with parchment. Arrange the fillets, skin-side down, on the parchment, then sprinkle the garlic slices over the fish. Top with the lemon slices followed by the Herbes Salées, then drizzle over the olive oil and sprinkle with black pepper.

3. Lift up the sides of the parchment paper, fold the edges together a few times to seal, and tuck the open ends under the fillets to enclose in a tight packet. Bake until the fish is just cooked through and flakes easily when poked with a fork, 8–12 minutes. Cool slightly, then slice open the parchment, taking care not to burn yourself as the steam escapes from the packet. Serve hot.

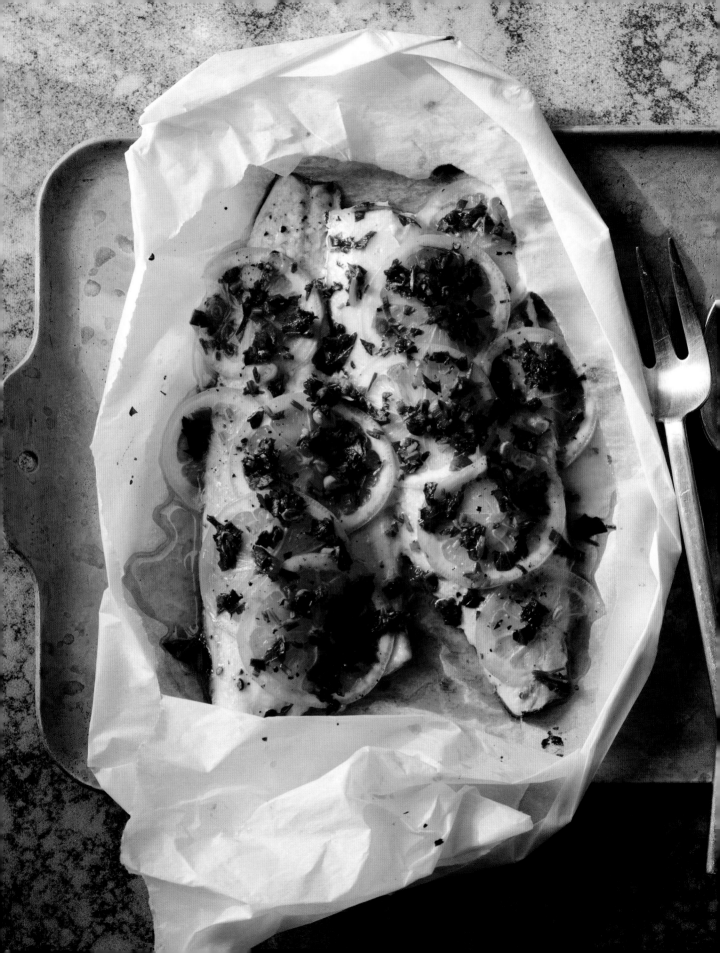

Pan-Seared Halibut with Barley-Artichoke Risotto

Serves 4

Total Time: 55 min.

FOR THE RISOTTO

1 Tbsp. extra-virgin olive oil

¾ cup pearl barley

1 medium yellow or white onion, finely chopped

1 garlic clove, finely chopped

¼ cup dry white wine

3 cups low-sodium chicken broth, hot

One 6-oz. jar marinated artichoke hearts, drained and coarsely chopped

1 cup fresh or frozen peas

¼ cup finely grated Parmesan cheese

2 tsp. Herbes Salées (page 117) (or substitute 1 tsp. finely chopped fresh parsley)

Kosher salt and freshly ground black pepper

FOR THE HALIBUT

Four 7-oz. halibut fillets

Kosher salt and freshly ground black pepper

½ tsp ground coriander (optional)

1 Tbsp. extra-virgin olive oil

1 Tbsp. Tomato Butter (page 122) (or substitute salted butter)

Artichokes are quite high in folate and fiber, but cleaning the spiny vegetable is awfully fiddly. If you like their peculiar, bittersweet and nutty flavor (we sure do!), then keep a jar or two of marinated artichoke hearts on hand. They're far superior in taste and texture to canned and frozen versions, and adding them to pastas, pizzas, and rice dishes is a quick way to elevate an everyday dish to a special meal.

If you have trouble finding halibut—or if you prefer a lower-cost alternative—swap it out for an equal portion of another thick, white-fleshed fish such as cod, haddock, or sea bass.

1. **Make the risotto:** In a medium pot, heat the oil over medium heat until it begins to shimmer. Add the barley and cook, stirring frequently, until fragrant and toasted, 2–3 minutes. Stir in the onions and garlic and continue cooking, stirring frequently, until the onions are softened, about 3 minutes. Add the wine and continue cooking, stirring continuously, until all of the liquid is absorbed, about 1 minute.

2. Begin adding the hot broth, ½ cup at a time, stirring continuously and allowing the liquid to absorb between additions. Cook just until the barley is almost tender (30–35 minutes, total). Stir in the artichoke hearts, peas, Parmesan, and Herbes Salées, then season to taste with salt and black pepper. Keep warm while you finish the fish.

3. Make the halibut: While the risotto cooks, pat the fillets dry with paper towels, then season all over with salt, black pepper, and coriander, if using. In a large heavy skillet, heat the oil over medium-high heat until it begins to shimmer. Add the fillets and cook without disturbing until the fish is lightly browned on the bottom and turning white and opaque about one-third of the way up from the skillet, 3–4 minutes. Gently flip the fillets (a wide, thin spatula is perfect for this), then continue cooking until the other side is lightly browned and turning white and opaque about one-third of the way up from the skillet, about 3 minutes more. Carefully transfer to a warm plate, dot with the Tomato Butter, then cover with an inverted bowl or aluminum foil and set aside in a warm place to finish steaming, about 2 minutes.

4. Divide the risotto among 4 wide bowls, top with the fish, and serve warm.

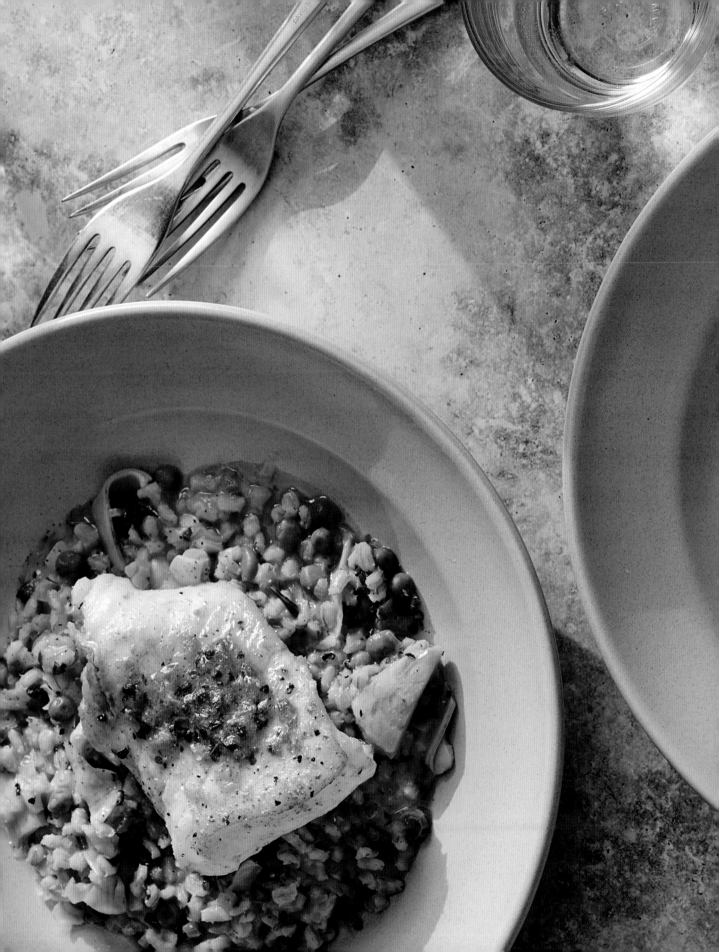

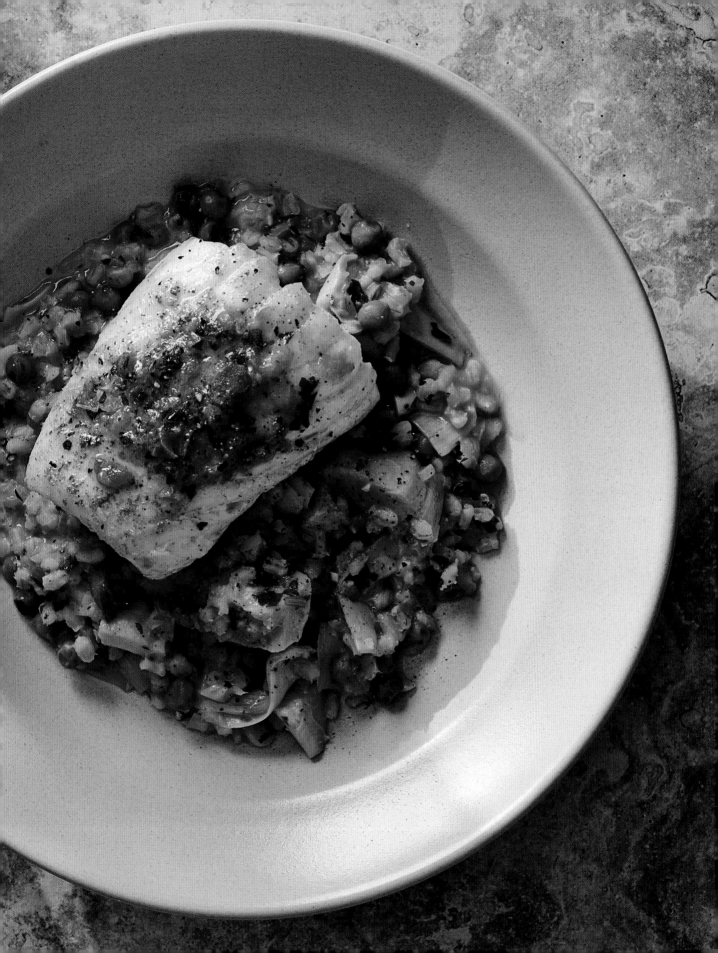

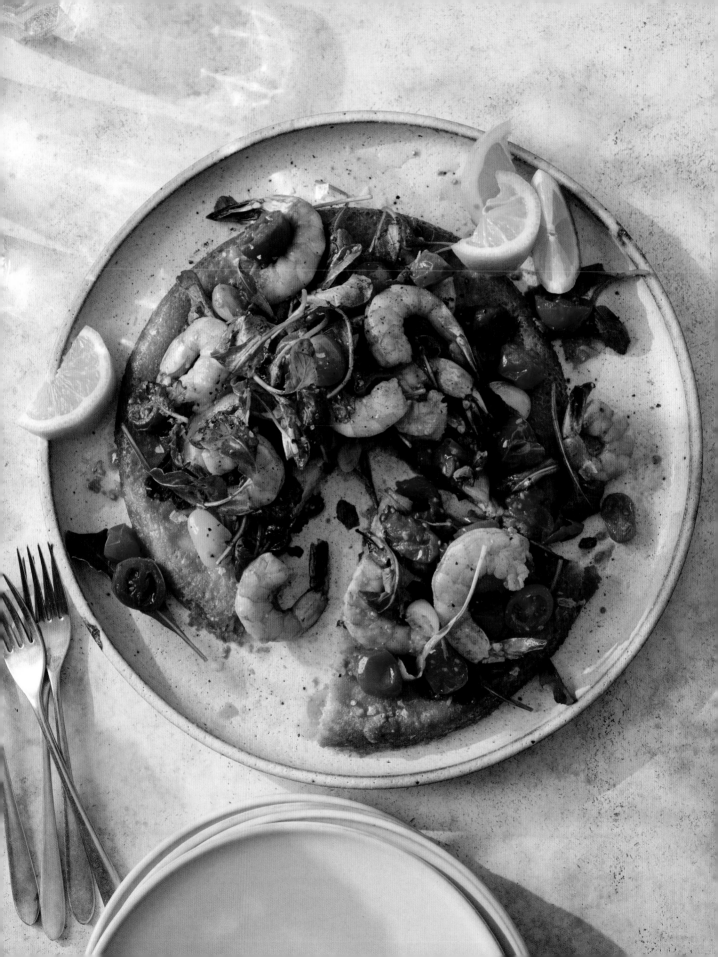

Savory Chickpea Pancake
with Shrimp, Saffron, and Arugula

Serves 4

Total Time: 1 hr. 30 min.

1 cup chickpea flour

¼ cup plus 1 Tbsp. extra-virgin olive oil, divided

2 garlic cloves, finely grated

¾ tsp. kosher salt, plus more as needed

Pinch of saffron, soaked in 1 Tbsp. warm water

16 medium shrimp (about ½ lb.), peeled and deveined

1 cup grape or cherry tomatoes, halved

1 tsp. finely grated lemon zest

¼ tsp. smoked paprika

1½ cups baby arugula

Lemon wedges, for serving

From Algeria and Spain's calentica to France's panisse and soca to Italy's farinata, olive oil–enriched chickpea pancakes abound. Our version is closest in texture and thickness to calentica, with a custardy texture somewhere between flan and polenta.

1. In a large bowl, whisk together the chickpea flour, 1 tablespoon of oil, garlic, salt, the saffron water, and 1½ cups of cold water. Cover with plastic wrap and set the batter aside at room temperature for at least 45 minutes and up to 24 hours.

2. Place a 10-inch cast-iron or oven-safe nonstick skillet on a rack in the center of the oven and preheat to 400°F. Set a second rack in the top third of the oven. When the skillet is hot, add 3 tablespoons of the oil, swirling carefully to coat the bottom surface. Return the skillet to the oven and let the oil heat for 2 minutes, then carefully pour in the chickpea batter (it will sizzle). Return the skillet to the oven once more and cook until the edges of the pancake are golden and a toothpick inserted into the center comes out clean, 20–25 minutes.

3. Meanwhile, on a large rimmed baking sheet, toss together the shrimp, tomatoes, remaining tablespoon of oil, lemon zest, and smoked paprika. Season lightly with salt, then transfer to the top rack of the oven and roast until the shrimp turn pink and are just cooked through and the tomatoes are starting to caramelize and sizzle, about 10 minutes.

4. Remove both the baking sheet and the skillet from the oven; let cool slightly. Using a thin spatula, loosen the pancake from the skillet, then invert onto a cutting board or large platter. Add the arugula to the baking sheet and toss with the shrimp and tomatoes to warm and wilt the greens slightly. Transfer the contents of the baking sheet to top the pancake. Cut into wedges and serve warm, with lemon wedges on the side, for squeezing.

Sesame-Ginger Broiled Salmon
with Asian Greens

| Serves 4 | Total Time: 20 min., plus 4 hr. marinating |

FOR THE SALMON

⅓ cup miso

2 Tbsp. rice vinegar

1 Tbsp. honey

1½ tsp. finely grated fresh ginger

1½ tsp. sesame oil

Four 6-oz. skin-on salmon fillets

FOR THE GREENS

1 tsp. vegetable oil

2 medium garlic cloves, thinly sliced

10 oz. (about 4 cups) bok choy, yu choy, water spinach, gai lan, or napa cabbage, sliced or torn into bite-sized pieces

1 tsp. low-sodium soy sauce

2 tsp. roasted sesame seeds, for garnish

2 cups steamed brown rice

This is a great prep-ahead dish. Once the salmon fillets are in the marinade, they keep well in the fridge for up to 24 hours. The flesh will flake away from the skin easily once the fillets are cooked through. Feel free to eat the crispy and omega-rich skin if you like.

1. **Make the salmon:** In a large bowl, whisk together the miso, vinegar, honey, ginger, and sesame oil. Add the salmon, turning to coat a few times, then cover tightly and refrigerate at least 4 and up to 24 hours.

2. When you're ready to cook the fish, preheat the oven to broil. Line a large rimmed baking sheet with foil. Remove the fillets from the bowl and use your hands to scrape off any excess marinade. Place the fillets, skin-side down, on the baking sheet, then broil until the fish is just cooked through, 6–8 minutes.

3. **Meanwhile, make the greens:** Heat the vegetable oil in a large skillet or wok over high heat, swirling to coat the inside surface. When the oil shimmers, add the garlic and cook, stirring continuously, until very fragrant but not yet colored, 30–60 seconds. Add the greens and 2 tablespoons of water and continue stir-frying until the leaves are bright green and wilted and the stems are tender, 6–8 minutes. Stir in the soy sauce, remove from heat, and divide among 4 dinner plates. Add a salmon fillet to each plate, garnish with sesame seeds, and serve with steamed brown rice on the side.

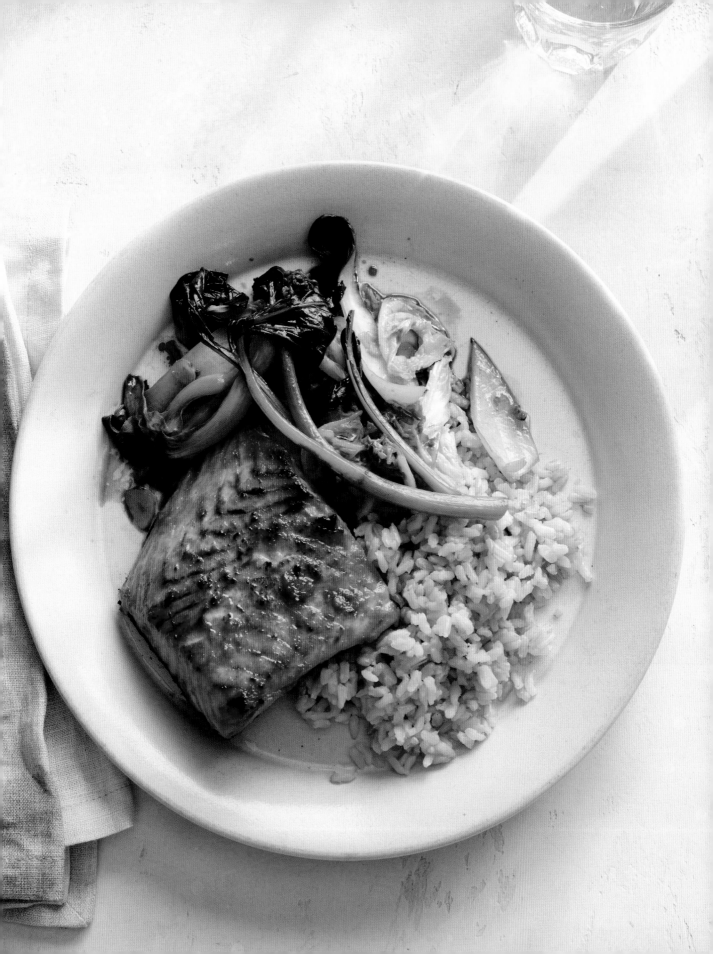

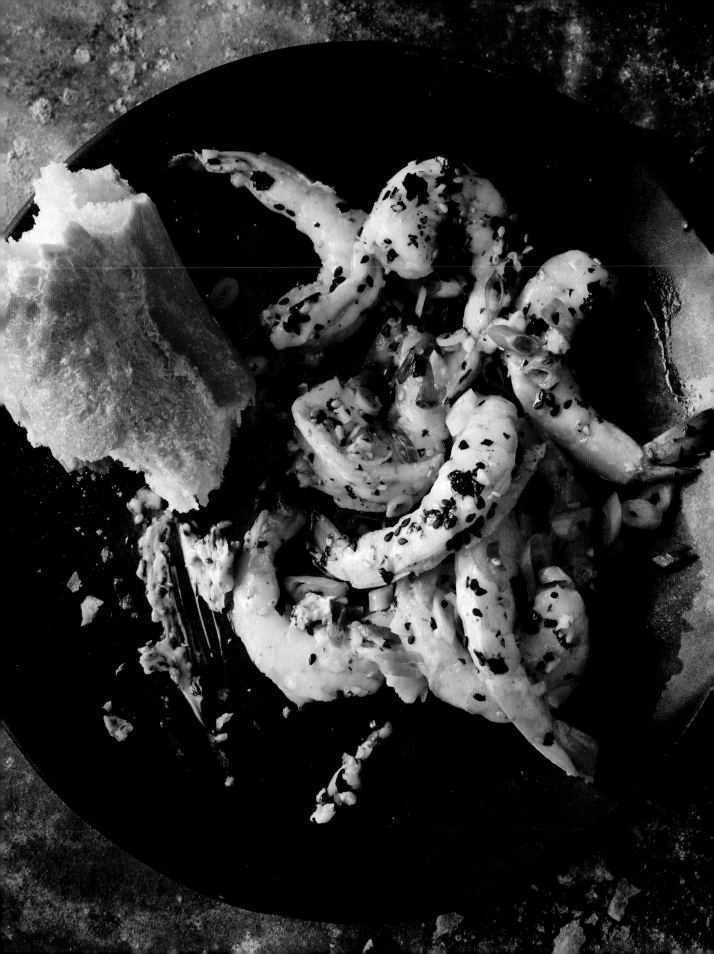

Garlic Shrimp
with Nori Butter and Lemon

Serves 4 | Total Time: 10 min.

1¼ lb. large shrimp,
peeled and deveined

1 Tbsp. extra-virgin olive oil

Kosher salt and freshly
ground black pepper

3 garlic cloves, finely chopped

2 Tbsp. Nori Butter (page 121)
(or substitute 1 Tbsp. salted
butter plus 1 tsp. sesame oil)

1 Tbsp. fresh lemon juice

2 tsp. black sesame seeds

4 scallions, trimmed
and thinly sliced

When you're in a hurry to get something on the dinner table fast, these quick-roasted shrimp are an excellent starting point loaded with sleep-supporting nutrients. Enjoy them with a simple salad or any sautéed green vegetable and some steamed rice, grits, or crusty bread for sopping up the flavorful and buttery juices.

1. Preheat the oven to 400°F. Place the shrimp on a large rimmed baking sheet, drizzle with the olive oil, and season lightly with salt and black pepper. Sprinkle the garlic over the top, then toss well to coat. Bake until the shrimp are cooked through and slightly browned at the edges, 5–7 minutes.

2. Remove the shrimp from the oven, then immediately dollop the Nori Butter over the top. Pour over the lemon juice and toss until the butter has melted and the shrimp are coated in the buttery sauce. Transfer to a platter, sprinkle with sesame seeds and scallions, and serve hot.

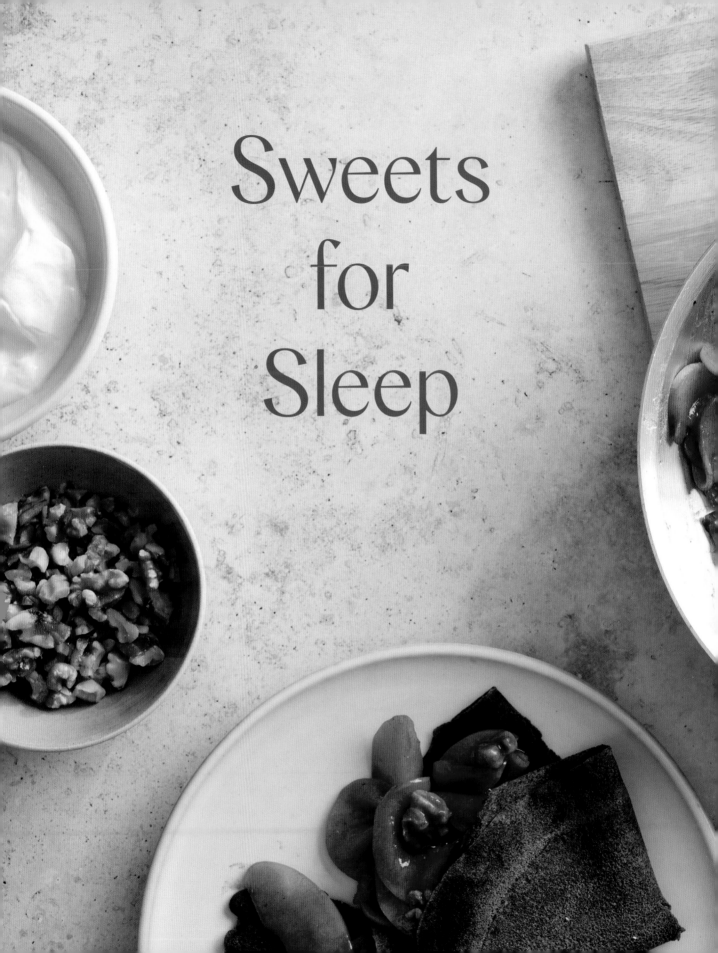

Sweets
for
Sleep

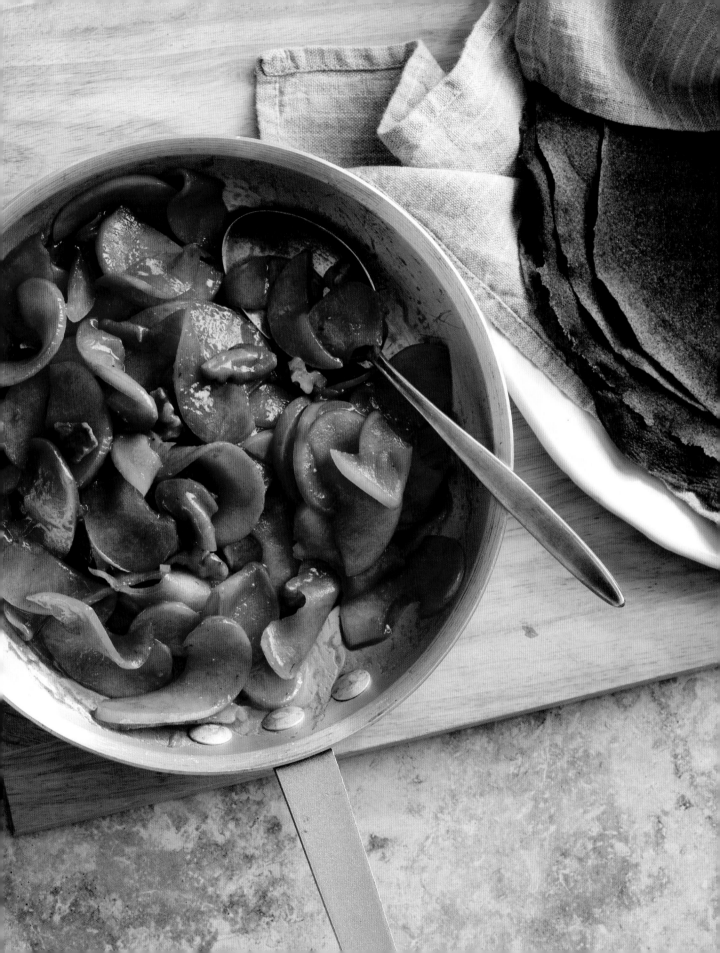

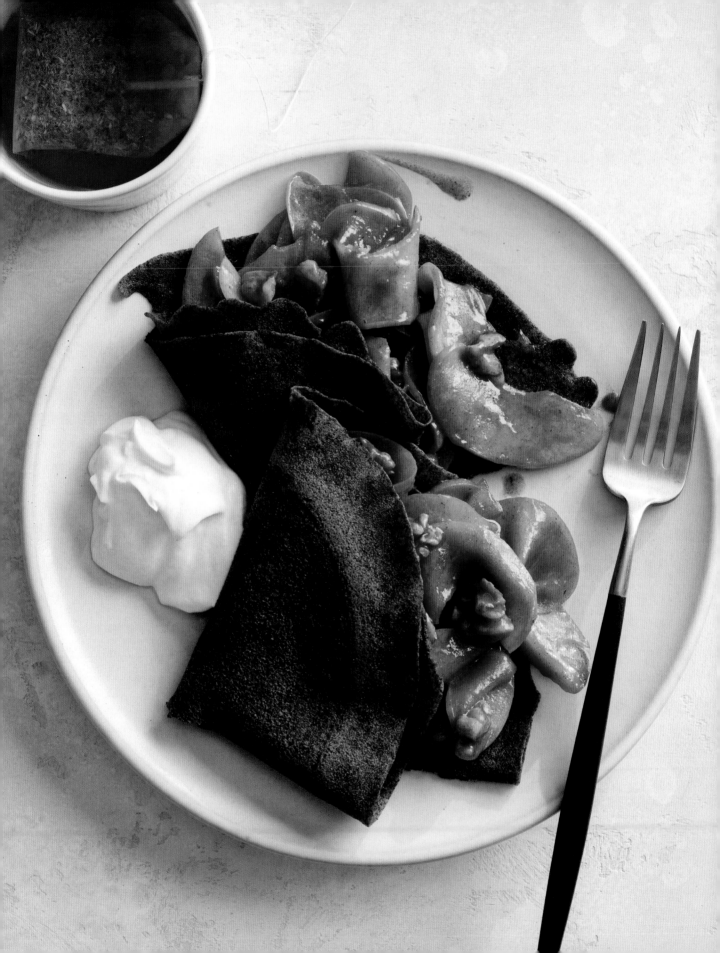

Buckwheat Crepes
with Apple-Walnut Filling

Serves 4	Total Time: 1 hr., plus 4 hr. resting the batter

FOR THE CREPES

1 cup (120 g) buckwheat flour

¼ cup molasses

1 large egg

¾ cup buttermilk

½ tsp. kosher salt

FOR THE APPLE-WALNUT FILLING

1 Tbsp. unsalted butter

1 Tbsp. almond oil (or substitute light olive oil), plus more for oiling the crepe pan

1 Tbsp. molasses

3 firm apples (such as Honeycrisp or Granny Smith), cored and thinly sliced (550 g)

2 tsp. cornstarch

¾ tsp. ground cinnamon

½ tsp. ground ginger

¼ tsp. ground nutmeg

Pinch of kosher salt

⅔ cup coarsely chopped walnuts, divided

¼ cup Greek yogurt, for serving (optional)

Marie-Pierre grew up eating buckwheat crepes in Quebec, Canada, and since the hearty grain is such a fantastic ingredient for supporting healthy sleep, we knew these paper-thin pancakes needed to have a place in our book. We decided to lightly sweeten them with a splash of nutrient-rich molasses, then fill them with spiced apple-walnut filling for an extra dose of melatonin and omega-3 fatty acids. Serve this dish as a sweet (but not-too-sweet) breakfast or lunch, or swap out the yogurt for ice cream and serve smaller portions for a cozy fall dessert.

The batter may be made ahead of time—it keeps well in the fridge for several days. We like to do just that and fire off a crepe or two as needed throughout the course of a week. The filling can be prepped in advance as well; microwave it for 30 to 60 seconds before using to rewarm.

1. **Make the crepes:** In a blender, combine the buckwheat flour, molasses, egg, buttermilk, and salt and blend until smooth. Transfer to a bowl or a liquid measuring cup, cover, and refrigerate for at least 4 hours or overnight.

2. **Shortly before you plan to cook the crepes, make the apple-walnut filling:** In a large skillet, heat butter and oil over medium heat until the butter begins to sputter. Stir in the molasses, then add the apples, cornstarch, cinnamon, ginger, nutmeg, and a pinch of salt. Cook, stirring occasionally, until the apples are just tender and the juices are bubbling and thickened, 12–14 minutes (if the apples do not release much liquid and the mixture is dry, stir in ¼–⅓ cup cool water and cook until the apples are tender and coated in a glossy sauce). Remove from heat, stir in half of the walnuts, and keep warm while you cook the crepes.

—continued—

3. Thin the crepe batter by whisking in ¼–½ cup cool water (it should have the consistency of a melted milkshake). Heat a large nonstick or well-seasoned carbon steel skillet (at least 9 inches) over medium heat. Soak a paper towel in oil and use it to very lightly grease the surface of the skillet. Pour a scant ¼ cup of the batter into the skillet, then immediately swirl to make a very thin pancake (pour any excess batter back into the bowl). Cook until the edges just barely begin to pull away from the sides of the skillet, 1–2 minutes, then use a thin spatula or your fingers to flip the crepe and cook until just set, about 30 seconds more. Turn the pancake out onto a heatproof plate and cover with a clean, dry kitchen towel while you continue cooking the rest of the batter, stacking the crepes atop each other as you go.

4. Fold 2 crepes in quarters and place on a plate. Tuck a quarter of the apple filling into the folds, sprinkle the crepes with chopped walnuts, and top with a tablespoon of yogurt, if using. Repeat with the remaining crepes (there should be 8 crepes total) and filling and serve warm.

Sesame Shortbread Cookies

Makes 26 cookies

Total Time: 40 min., plus 2 hr. chilling the dough

8 Tbsp. softened unsalted butter

½ cup (60 g) powdered sugar, sifted

½ cup tahini (125 g)

1½ cups (185 g) all-purpose flour

⅓ cup (45 g) whole wheat flour

1 Tbsp. cornstarch

1 tsp. kosher salt

½ cup sesame seeds

Tryptophan-rich tahini gives these tender little biscuits an almost peanut buttery flavor. We like them in the afternoon or after dinner, paired with decaf coffee or a cup of mint tea. When stored at room temperature, butter shortbread ages beautifully, improving in both flavor and texture. Make a batch at the beginning of the month, and enjoy them for weeks.

1. In the bowl of a stand mixer fitted with the paddle attachment, beat the butter, powdered sugar, and tahini on medium until smooth, 2–4 minutes. Add the flours, cornstarch, and salt and continue mixing, scraping the bottom and sides of the bowl once or twice, just until homogenous. (Alternatively, this may be mixed in a large bowl using an electric hand mixer.)

2. Line a baking sheet with parchment. Pour the sesame seeds into a wide bowl. Scoop the dough into 26 pieces (about 1 packed tablespoon each). Roll one piece into a ball, then drop it into the bowl of sesame seeds and roll it around, pressing to adhere the seeds. Place the ball on the parchment and flatten into a ½-inch-thick disk. Continue rolling and shaping all of the dough in this manner, then transfer the sheet to the fridge until the cookies are firm, at least 2 hours. (If storing raw cookies longer than 4 hours in the fridge, cover tightly with plastic wrap.)

3. When you are ready to bake the cookies, position a rack in the center of the oven and preheat it to 325°F. Arrange the chilled cookies on the lined sheet, leaving at least 1 inch between each one. Bake, turning once halfway through cooking, until the seeds are just beginning to brown along the bottoms of the cookies and the top surfaces look dry and slightly cracked (the cookies will still be soft), 16–18 minutes. Cool completely before serving. Store any leftovers in an airtight container at room temperature for up to 2 weeks.

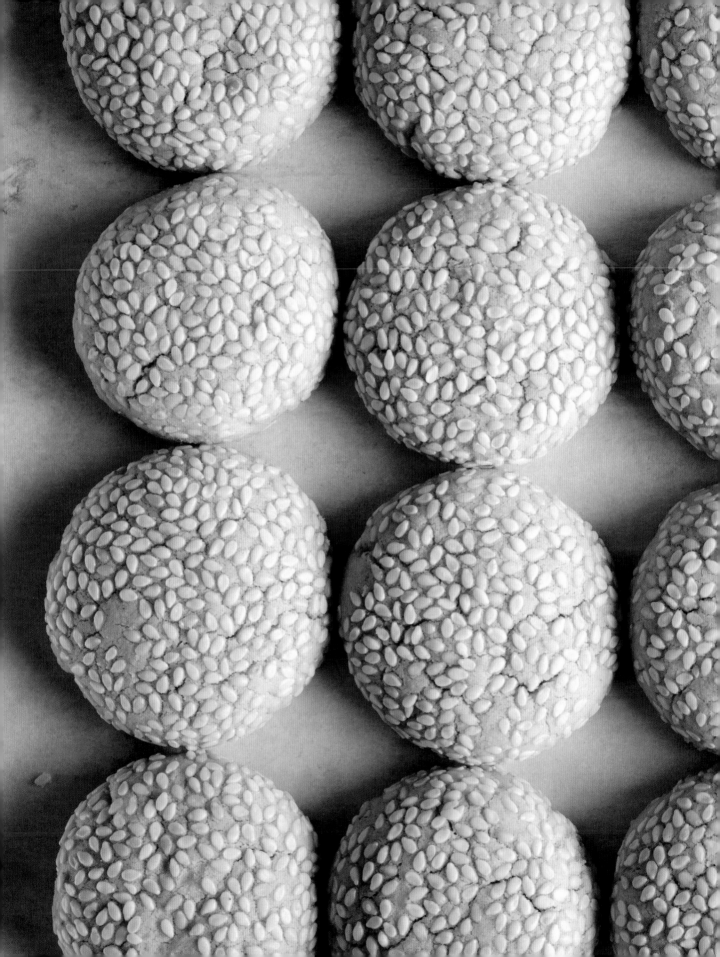

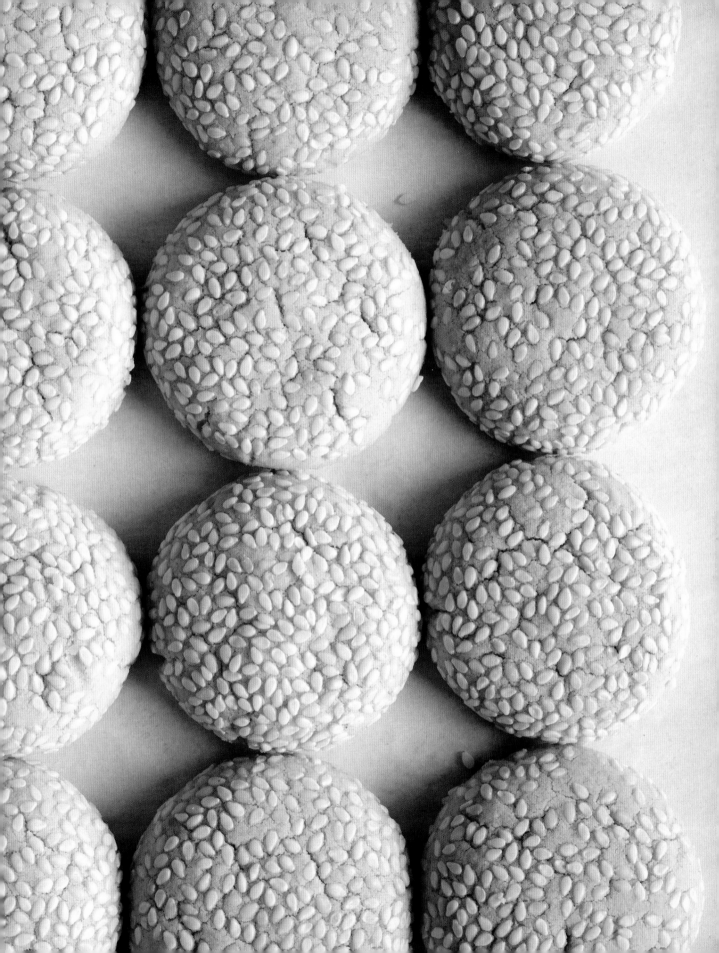

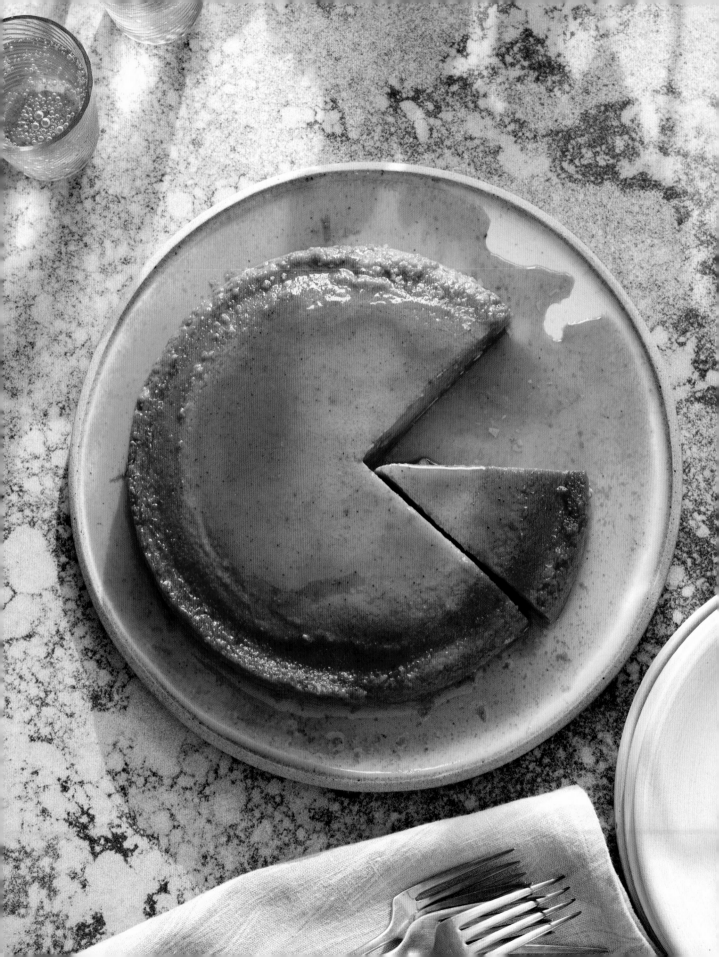

Maple-Pumpkin Crème Caramel

Serves 8–10

Total Time: 1 hr. 45 min., plus 12 hr. to chill the custard

FOR THE MAPLE-CARAMEL LAYER

¼ cup sugar

½ cup maple syrup

¼ tsp. flaky sea salt

FOR THE PUMPKIN CUSTARD

One 15-oz. can pumpkin purée

One 14-oz. can sweetened condensed milk

1½ cups milk

4 large eggs

1 Tbsp. vanilla extract

1½ tsp. ground cinnamon

½ tsp. freshly grated nutmeg

¼ tsp. ground clove

Marie-Pierre comes from Quebec and has a particular fondness for maple syrup—which also happens to have a fairly low glycemic index compared to other sweeteners—so we added it to the caramel for this delicate custard. Don't be alarmed when the caramel layer does not firm up in the pan; just pour the custard base gently to avoid sloshing as much as possible and trust that it will unmold beautifully. The appealing pumpkin-spice flavor profile of this dessert is reminiscent of holiday pumpkin pie, minus the buttery crust.

1. **Make the maple-caramel layer:** In a medium, heavy pot, combine the sugar and 1 tablespoon of water. Bring to a boil over medium-high heat, then cook without stirring but rotating the pot occasionally to distribute the heat evenly, until the mixture turns a light golden brown, 2–3 minutes. Watch carefully—sugar can burn quickly. Remove from heat and stir in the maple syrup until combined with the sugar mixture (if the caramel seizes up, return the pot to low heat if needed to remelt). Pour the maple-caramel into an 8-inch round cake pan, sprinkle with the flaky salt, then set aside to cool for at least 30 minutes (the syrup will form a skin but will not set completely).

2. Meanwhile, position a rack in the center of the oven and preheat it to 350°F.

3. **Make the pumpkin custard:** In a large bowl, whisk together the pumpkin purée, condensed milk, milk, eggs, vanilla, cinnamon, nutmeg, and clove until completely smooth. Place a fine-mesh sieve in a large, spouted measuring cup or bowl, then pass the custard through it, pressing any solids through with a silicone spatula. Gently pour the custard over the cooked maple caramel. (Avoid sloshing to prevent the cooked maple caramel from mixing with the

—continued—

custard.) Place the cake pan in a roasting pan large enough to hold it flat, then fill the roasting pan with hot tap water to come two-thirds up the sides of the cake pan. Cover tightly with foil or a large baking sheet, then carefully bake until the custard is just set, 65–70 minutes. (It will be firm but still jiggly in the middle; a knife inserted into the center will come out clean.) Remove from the water bath, place on a wire rack, and cool to room temperature. Cover with plastic wrap and refrigerate for at least 12 and up to 24 hours.

4. When ready to serve, uncover the custard and run a thin knife around the edge. Place a large, flat serving plate over the cake pan and quickly and confidently invert. Place the plate on a flat surface (you should hear the custard release and plop onto the plate), then remove the cake pan, allowing the maple sauce to run out over the top of the custard. Cut into wedges and serve cold.

Roasted Figs
with Walnuts and Greek Yogurt

Serves 2

Total Time: 25 min.

1 Tbsp. plus 1 tsp. extra-virgin olive oil, divided

14 fresh figs, stemmed and halved

5 bay leaves (fresh or dried)

1 Tbsp. coarsely chopped walnuts

1½ tsp. honey or maple syrup

2 tsp. fresh lemon juice

Pinch of flaky sea salt

¼ cup Greek yogurt

Kat learned to make this dish from cookbook author Kate Hill, who operates a cooking school in southwestern France. The bay laurel tree in Hill's garden was the inspiration for this simple-yet-elegant and fragrant dish. If you like, substitute the Greek yogurt for any other cultured fresh cheese like fromage blanc, quark, or farmers' cheese.

1. Position a rack in the center of the oven and preheat it to 400°F.

2. Lightly oil a small skillet or shallow baking dish with 1 teaspoon of the oil, then arrange the figs, cut-side up, in a single layer. Tuck the bay leaves between the fig halves, sprinkle with walnuts, then drizzle evenly with the honey and the remaining tablespoon of oil. Roast until the juices are bubbling and syrupy and the figs are softened, 10–12 minutes. Cool slightly, then remove and discard the bay leaves.

3. Divide the figs and their cooking juices among 2 dessert plates. Drizzle with lemon juice, top with a pinch of flaky sea salt, and serve warm, with a dollop of yogurt.

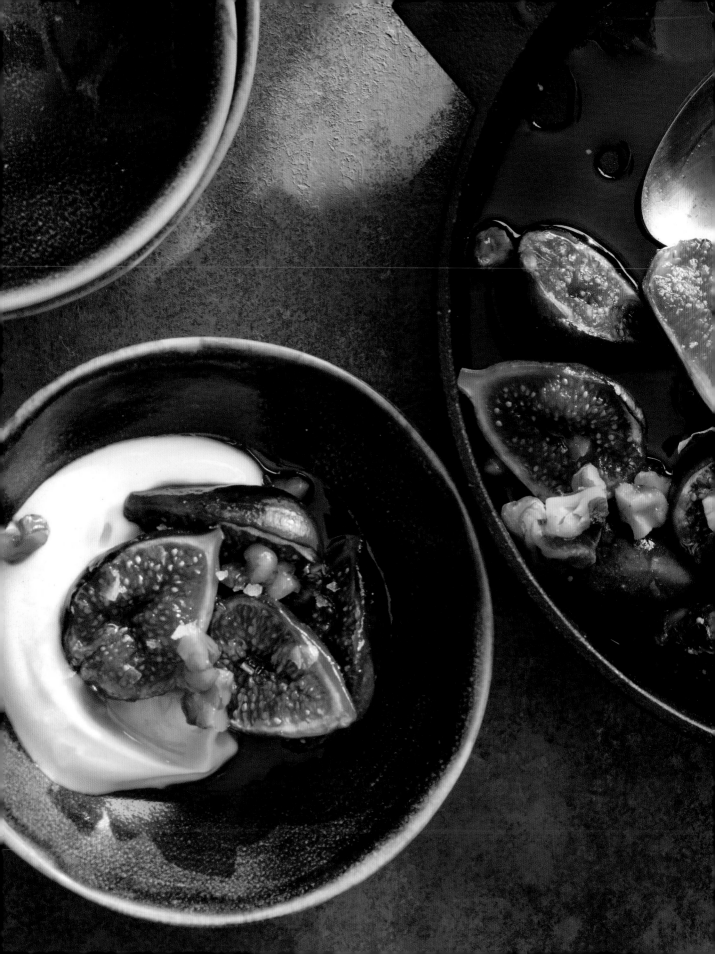

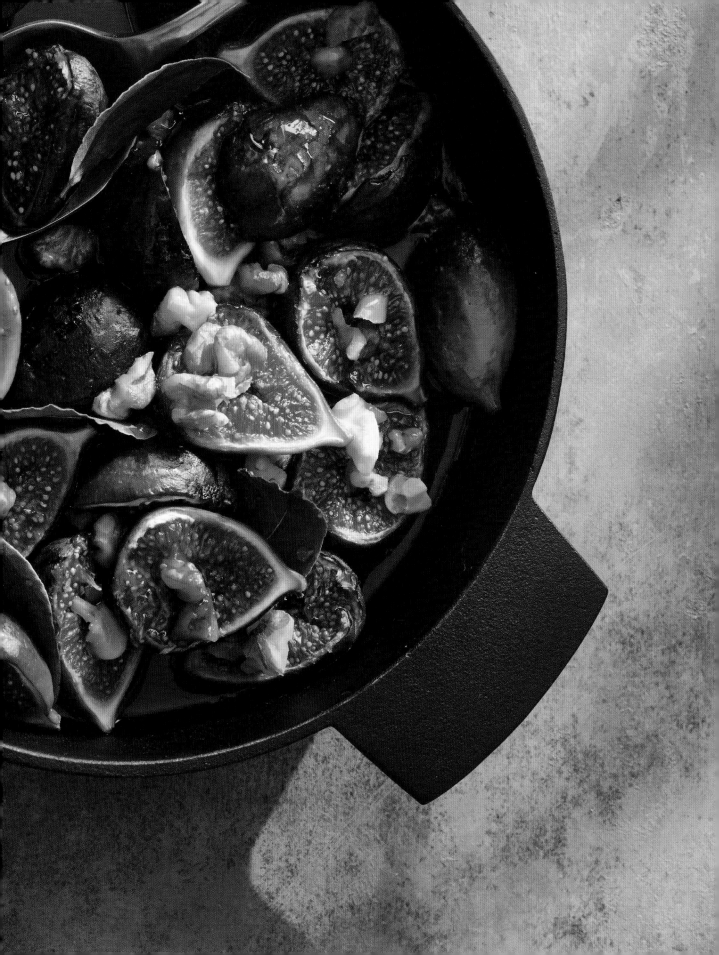

Plantain Cake
with Yogurt–Cream Cheese Frosting

Serves 12	Total Time: 1 hr. 15 min.

FOR THE CAKE

Nonstick baking spray

1 cup (120 g) whole wheat flour

½ cup (70 g) all-purpose flour

1¼ tsp. baking powder

½ tsp. baking soda

1 tsp. ground ginger

½ tsp. ground cinnamon

¼ tsp. ground nutmeg

1 tsp. kosher salt

2 very ripe plantains, peeled and mashed (325 g)

2 large eggs

⅓ cup unsulfured molasses

⅔ cup coconut milk

FOR THE FROSTING

⅔ cup light cream cheese, softened

¼ cup powdered sugar

⅓ cup plain Greek yogurt

1 tsp. vanilla extract

This recipe is exceptionally high in zinc, one of the essential minerals connected to the body's melatonin and serotonin production. Coconut milk lends a faint tropical note, which we love, but feel free to swap it out for oat, nut, or even cow's milk if you prefer. Wrapped tightly in plastic, this cake freezes very well, so don't hesitate to make it in advance, whenever your plantains hit peak ripeness. It also lasts in the refrigerator for a week after baking. Hold off on mixing the frosting and adding it to the cake until you are ready to serve.

1. **Make the cake:** Preheat the oven to 350°F. Lightly grease an 8- by 4-inch loaf pan with nonstick baking spray.

2. In a large bowl, whisk the flours, the baking powder, baking soda, ginger, cinnamon, nutmeg, and salt. In a medium bowl, whisk the mashed plantains, eggs, molasses, and coconut milk. Fold the wet ingredients into the flour mixture until just combined, then transfer to the loaf pan. Smooth the surface of the cake with a spatula or the back of a spoon, then bake until a toothpick inserted in the center comes out clean, 40–45 minutes. Cool completely to room temperature in the loaf pan before unmolding.

3. **Meanwhile, make the frosting:** In a medium bowl, whisk the cream cheese until smooth. Sift the powdered sugar into the bowl and whisk to combine, then whisk in the yogurt and vanilla extract until very smooth.

4. Once the cake is completely cooled, run a thin knife along the edge of the pan to unmold. Using an offset spatula or the back of a spoon, spread the frosting evenly over the top surface in swoops and swishes. Cut into slices and serve at room temperature.

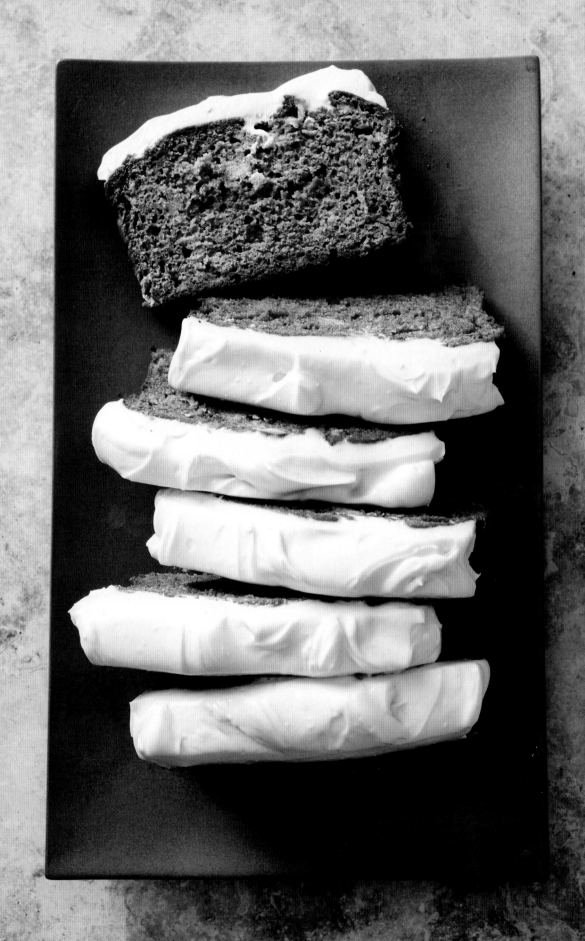

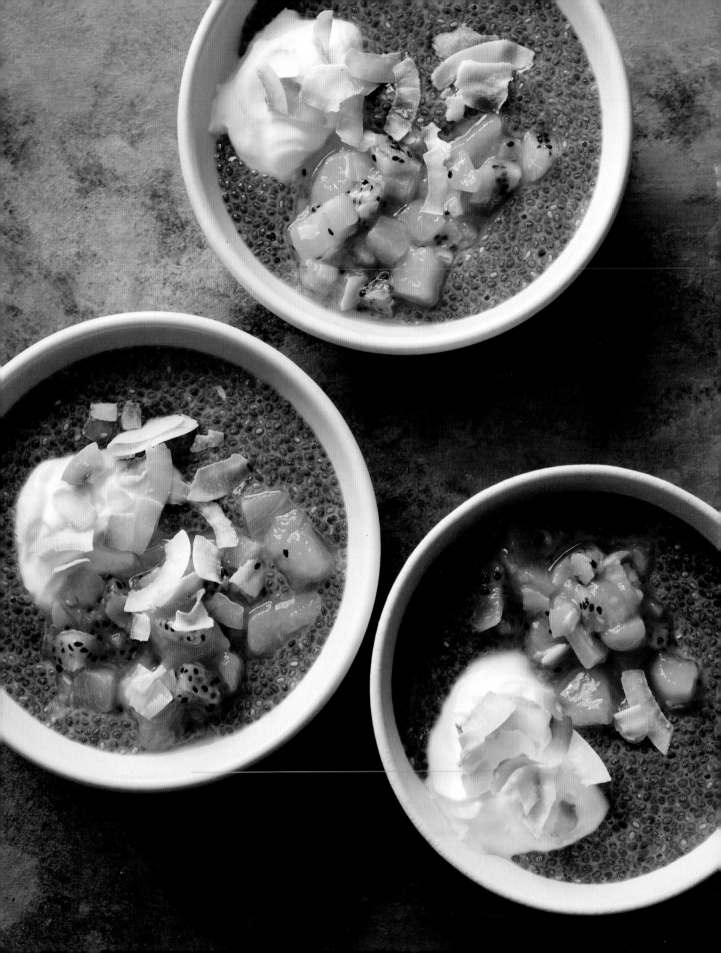

Chia Pudding
with Tropical Fruit Compote and Greek Yogurt

| Serves 4 | Total Time: 15 min., plus 4 hr. for the pudding to set |

2 cups milk or unsweetened rice, oat, or almond milk

½ cup chia seeds

3 Tbsp. maple syrup or honey

½ tsp. vanilla or almond extract

Pinch of kosher salt

¾ cups Tropical Fruit Compote (page 101)

¾ cup Greek yogurt

¼ cup toasted coconut flakes or sliced almonds

Teeny-tiny chia seeds are a sleep-supporting superfood. They're not only rich in protein and tryptophan; they also provide a ton of omega-3 and omega-6 fatty acids and are rich in magnesium, fiber, complex carbohydrates, vitamin B_6, and zinc. Their unique ability to absorb water makes them a fun pantry addition: Add them to smoothies and sauces to act as a thickening agent and emulsifier, or use them as a base for this refreshing summer pudding. You can exchange the Tropical Fruit Compote in this recipe for the Midsummer Compote (page 98) or Winter Compote (page 100).

1. In a medium bowl, whisk together the milk, chia seeds, maple syrup, vanilla, and salt. Set aside at room temperature for 10 minutes, then whisk again to redistribute the seeds, breaking up any clumps that have formed. Cover and refrigerate for at least 4 and up to 36 hours.

2. To serve, divide the chia pudding among 4 ramekins or dessert bowls. Top with compote, yogurt, and coconut flakes and serve cold.

Easy Stone Fruit Sorbet

Serves 4

Total Time: 10 min., plus 3 hr. for freezing the sorbet

1½ cups Midsummer Compote (page 98)

1 Tbsp. honey or maple syrup

Lightly cooked and puréed fresh fruit makes an excellent and healthful sorbet base. Not all home cooks have an ice cream maker, so we developed this no-churn recipe using our gingery Midsummer Compote. The technique also works with the Tropical Fruit Compote (page 101); just increase the sweetener to 3 tablespoons to ensure it refreezes soft enough to scoop.

1. In a blender or food processor, combine the compote and honey and blend until smooth. Transfer to a nonreactive baking dish or wide plastic container (rectangular plastic takeout containers work great for this), then freeze until solid, about 3 hours.

2. When the purée is completely frozen, use a fork to break it into pieces, then transfer the pieces back to the blender. Blend again until smooth, then scoop the sorbet into a chilled bowl and serve. For a firmer texture, transfer the sorbet back to the container, cover, and freeze until firm, at least 30 minutes.

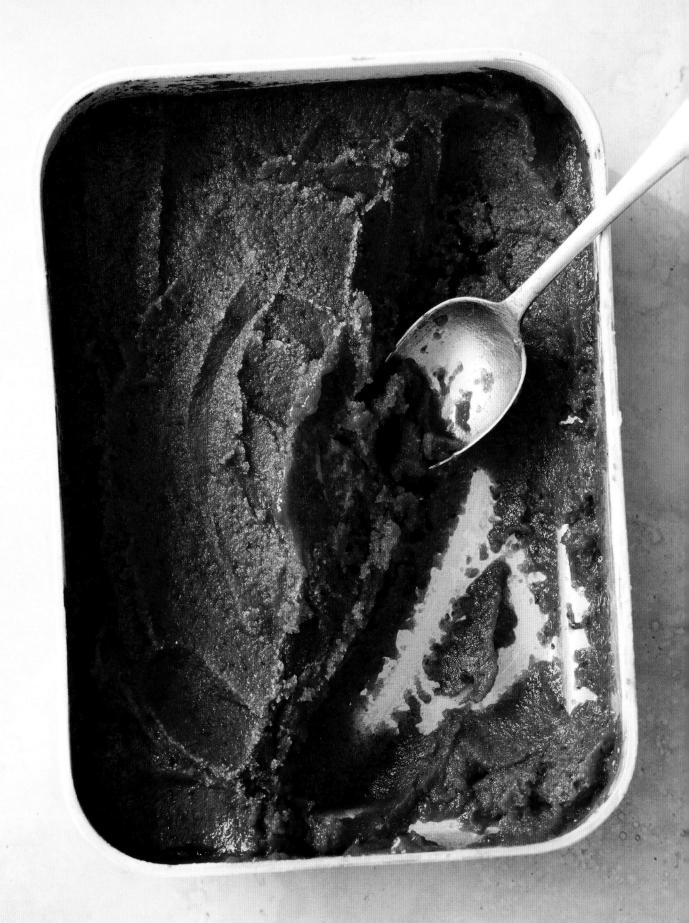

Banana-Chamomile Shortcake

| Serves 12 | Total Time: 40 min. |

FOR THE OAT BISCUITS

Nonstick baking spray

1½ cups (204 g) all-purpose flour, plus more for dusting

1 cup (138 g) whole wheat flour

1 cup (100 g) rolled (old-fashioned) oats

1 Tbsp. plus ½ tsp. baking powder

1¼ tsp. baking soda

1¼ tsp. kosher salt

⅓ cup olive oil or almond-olive oil blend

1 cup buttermilk, plus more for brushing

FOR SERVING

¾ cup Chamomile-Ginger Cordial (page 267) (or substitute ½ cup brewed chamomile tea stirred with ¼ cup honey)

1½ cups Greek yogurt

2 cups Honey-Butter Bananas (page 103)

⅓ cup sliced almonds (optional)

This cozy shortcake recipe may be adapted to substitute any of the other melatonin-rich fruit compotes in this book for the Honey-Butter Bananas. You could also use a handful of in-season berries or sliced stone fruit. The oat-laden drop biscuits are rich in tryptophan and fiber, and they may be assembled ahead of time and frozen before baking. If finishing the biscuits out of the freezer, allow them to thaw in the fridge for 1 hour before transferring to the oven.

1. Position a rack in the center of the oven and preheat it to 400°F. Lightly oil a 10-inch cast-iron skillet with nonstick baking spray or olive oil and set aside.

2. **Make the oat biscuits:** In a large bowl, whisk together the flours, oats, baking powder, baking soda, and salt. Add the olive oil and, using your hands, rub it into the dry ingredients until the mixture begins to clump together and looks like coarse, wet sand. Add the buttermilk, then incorporate the liquid into the dry ingredients by tossing the mixture gently with your fingers and palms facing upward, just until a shaggy dough forms.

3. Using a large cookie scoop or a ¼-cup measuring cup, divide the dough into 12 even balls. (Don't pack the dough too hard into the scoop or the biscuit will be dense.) Transfer the biscuits to the skillet (the sides will touch lightly), then brush the tops lightly with buttermilk and bake until the tops are lightly golden brown, 20–25 minutes.

4. To serve, split the biscuits in half crosswise. Place the bottom of biscuit on a small dessert plate. Drizzle with a tablespoon of the Chamomile–Ginger Cordial, then spread with a scant 2 tablespoons of yogurt. Add a scant 3 tablespoons of Honey-Butter Bananas, followed by the biscuit top. Garnish with another small dollop of yogurt and a pinch of sliced almonds, if using. Repeat with the remaining biscuits and fillings and serve warm or at room temperature.

Blackberry-Plum Galette with a Corn Crust

Serves 6

Total Time: 1 hr. 20 min.

FOR THE DOUGH

⅔ cup (78 g) all-purpose flour, plus more for dusting

⅓ cup (42 g) whole wheat flour

¼ cup (30 g) cornmeal

1 Tbsp. sugar

¼ tsp. kosher salt

¼ cup coconut oil, solid but soft

FOR THE FILLING

7 medium plums, pitted and sliced ½ in. thick (520 g)

⅓ cup maple syrup

2 Tbsp. cornstarch

1 tsp. vanilla or almond extract

1 tsp. ground ginger

½ tsp. kosher salt

1 cup (135 g) blackberries

While coconut oil, a plant-based tropical oil, is high in saturated fats, the majority of those are medium-chain fatty acids (MCFAs), which do not adversely affect cardiovascular health like the long-chain fatty acid prevalent in animal-derived fats do. We find it also makes a lovely vegan pie crust.

Coconut oil liquefies at warm room temperature, so be sure it is cool enough to solidify (but not so cold that it is unmalleable) when you make this flaky pastry dough.

1. **Make the dough:** In a large bowl, combine the flours, cornmeal, sugar, and salt. Add the coconut oil in spoonfuls, then rub the oil into the dry ingredients using your hands until it has the consistency of a coarse meal. Add 2 tablespoons of ice water and continue working the mixture between your hands just until a shaggy dough forms, adding more ice water, a drizzle at a time (up to 2 additional tablespoons), if the dough is too crumbly to hold together when squeezed. Transfer the dough to a sheet of plastic wrap, flatten to a ½-inch-thick disk, then wrap tightly and set aside at cool room temperature for 15 minutes. (Don't refrigerate or freeze this dough.)

2. **Meanwhile make the filling:** Meanwhile, in a large bowl, gently toss the plums with the maple syrup, cornstarch, vanilla, ginger, and salt.

3. Preheat the oven to 400°F. Lightly flour a large sheet of parchment paper and place it on a large work surface. Unwrap the dough, place it on the floured parchment paper, lightly dust the surface of the dough with flour, then roll the dough to an 11-inch circle. Lift the sides of the parchment paper to carefully slide both it and the dough round onto a large rimmed baking sheet.

4. Gently toss the berries into the plum mixture, then mound the fruit filling in the center of the dough, leaving a 2-inch border all around. Fold up the edges of the pastry to partially cover the filling, then drizzle any juices that remain in the bowl over the fruit. Bake until the pastry is golden brown, the plums are softened, and the juices are bubbling and thickened, 35–40 minutes.

5. Allow the galette to cool slightly, then slide a thin spatula under it to detach it from the parchment paper. Slide onto a wide, flat plate, cut into wedges, and serve warm or at room temperature.

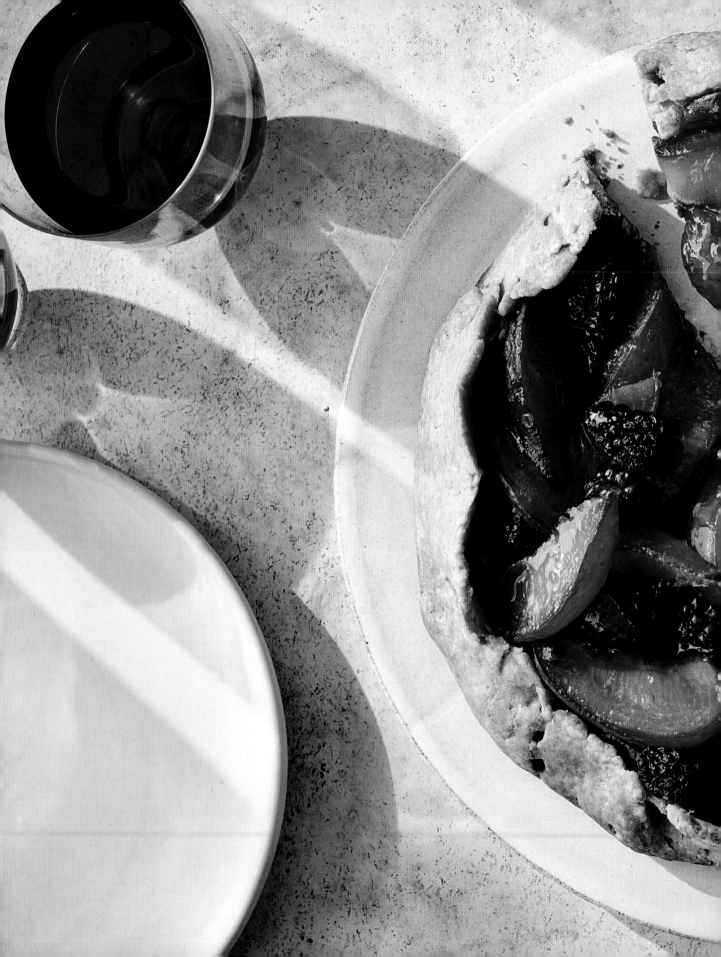

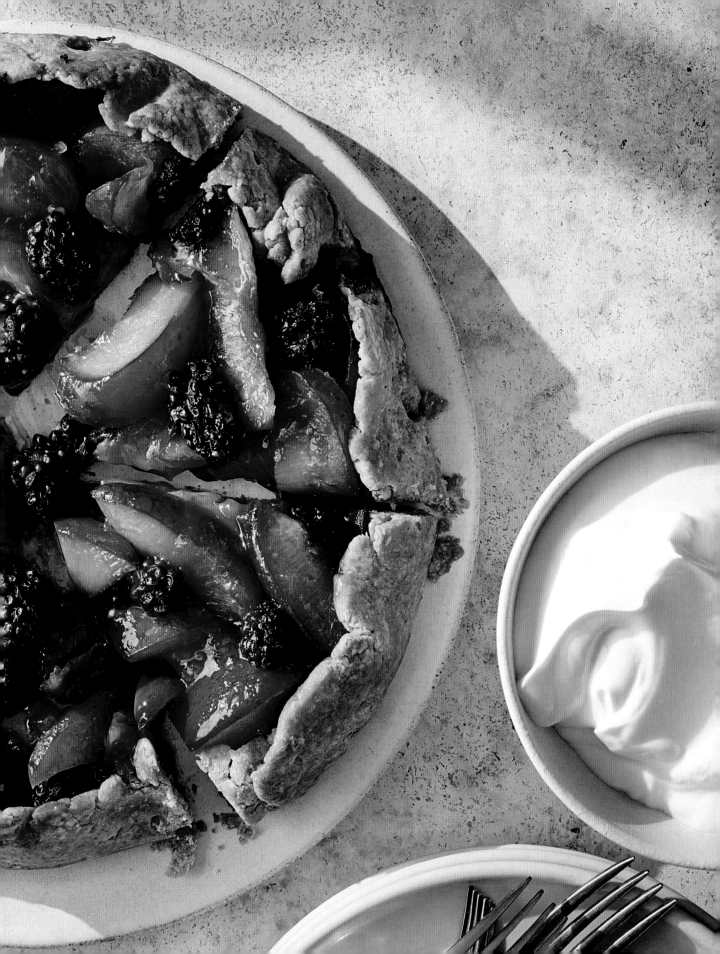

Brown Rice Pudding
with Saffron, Dates, and Pistachios

Serves 4–6

Total Time: 1 hr. 10 min., plus 4 hr. for chilling the pudding

¾ cup brown rice

¼ tsp. kosher salt

1 cinnamon stick (optional)

2 cups unsweetened rice, oat, or almond milk, divided

Pinch of saffron threads, soaked in 1 Tbsp. warm water

3 Tbsp. honey

¼ tsp. ground cardamom

1 large egg

8 medium dates, pitted and torn or sliced into bite-sized pieces (about ½ cup)

¼ tsp. rosewater

¼ tsp. vanilla extract

¼ cup plus 2 Tbsp. coarsely chopped roasted pistachios

Dried rose petals, for garnish (optional)

Dates with pits tend to be far softer and more tender than packaged pitted types, so it's worth the small amount of effort involved to pit them yourself. If, however, you can only find pitted dates, don't worry—just soak them in some warm water or black tea while you make this Persian-inspired pudding, then drain them right before using. If you don't like the fragrance of rosewater, feel free to swap it out for orange blossom water, or even a few extra drops of vanilla or almond extract.

1. In a medium pot, combine the rice, salt, cinnamon stick, if using, and 1½ cups of cold water. Bring to a boil over medium-high heat, then cover, lower the heat, and cook until all of the water is absorbed, about 40 minutes.

2. Uncover the cooked rice, remove the cinnamon stick, then stir in 1½ cups of the milk, the saffron water, the honey, and cardamom. Set over medium heat and cook, stirring frequently, until very creamy, about 15 minutes.

3. In a medium bowl, whisk together the remaining ½ cup of milk and the egg until combined, then stir the egg-milk mixture and the dates into the rice pot. Cook, stirring continuously and scraping the bottom of the pot with a silicone spatula, until the pudding is slightly thickened, about 2 minutes more. (Don't overcook or the egg may scramble.) Remove from heat and stir in the rosewater and vanilla.

4. Transfer the pudding into dessert bowls or a large serving bowl, cover, and refrigerate until chilled, at least 4 hours. Serve cold, topped with chopped pistachios and dried rose petals, if using.

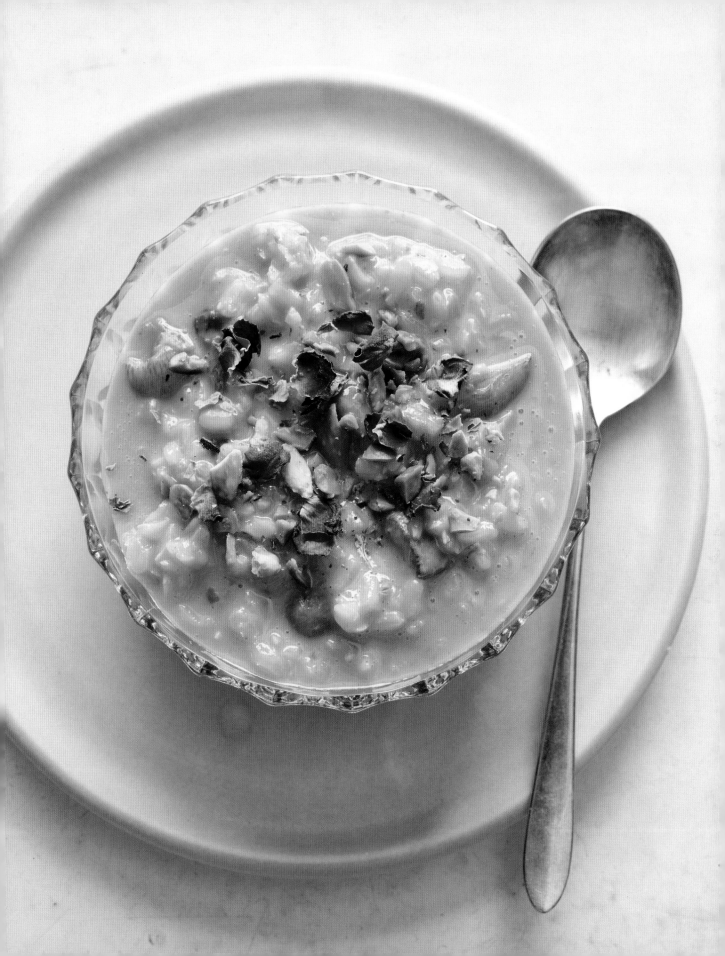

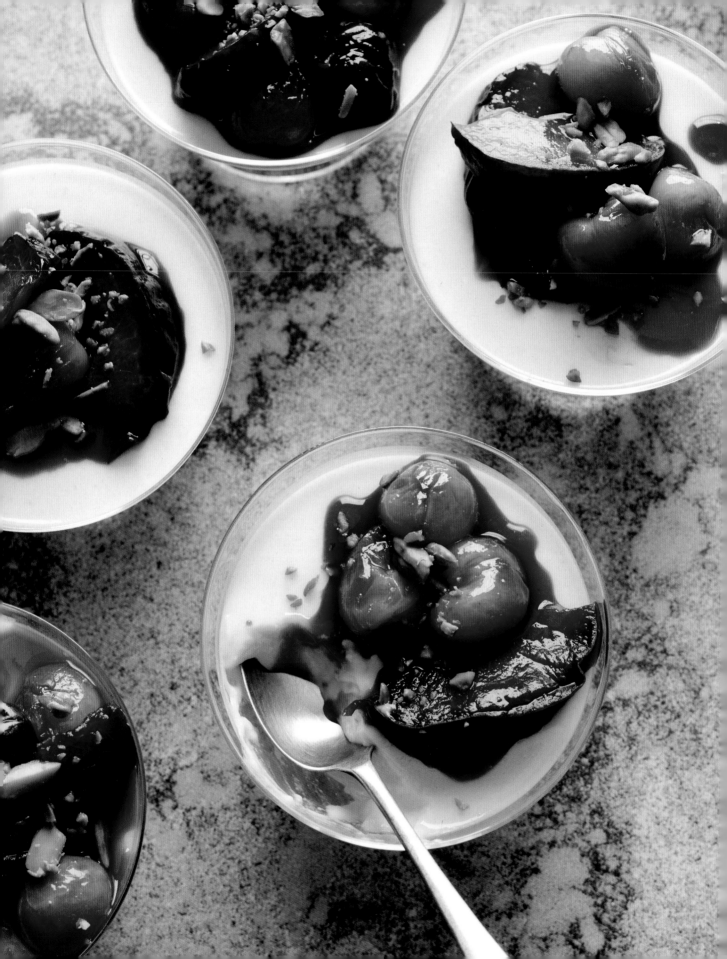

Chamomile-Ginger Panna Cotta
with Midsummer Compote and Pistachios

Serves 6 | Total Time: 20 min., plus 3 hr. for the panna cotta to set

1 cup Chamomile-Ginger Cordial (page 267) (or substitute ⅔ cup chamomile or ginger tea plus ⅓ cup honey), divided

One 8-g packet plain powdered gelatin

2 cups plain kefir (or substitute plain [not Greek] yogurt)

1½ tsp. vanilla extract

½ cup Midsummer Compote (page 98), Winter Compote (page 100), or Tropical Fruit Compote (page 101)

1 Tbsp. plus 1 tsp. coarsely chopped pistachios

Kefir—pronounced kee-feer—is a tangy, fermented dairy beverage that originated in the North Caucasus region, and is now widely available in North America. Like yogurt, kefir is loaded with live active cultures that improve the gut microbiome. A 2019 study showed that postmenopausal women showed improvements in insomnia after drinking 2 cups of kefir a day for a month. We find it makes a tasty base for these jiggly, eggless custards.

1. In a small bowl, sprinkle the gelatin powder over ¼ cup of the Chamomile-Ginger Cordial. Set aside until the powder is fully hydrated, about 5 minutes.

2. Meanwhile, in a small pot, heat the remaining ¾ cup of cordial over medium heat until it begins to simmer. Remove from heat and whisk in the bloomed gelatin mixture until it has fully dissolved. Whisk in the kefir and vanilla, then strain through a fine-mesh sieve into 6 ramekins or small bowls. Cover loosely with plastic wrap and refrigerate until fully set, at least 3 and up to 48 hours.

3. Top each panna cotta with a scoop of compote and a sprinkle of pistachios. Serve cold.

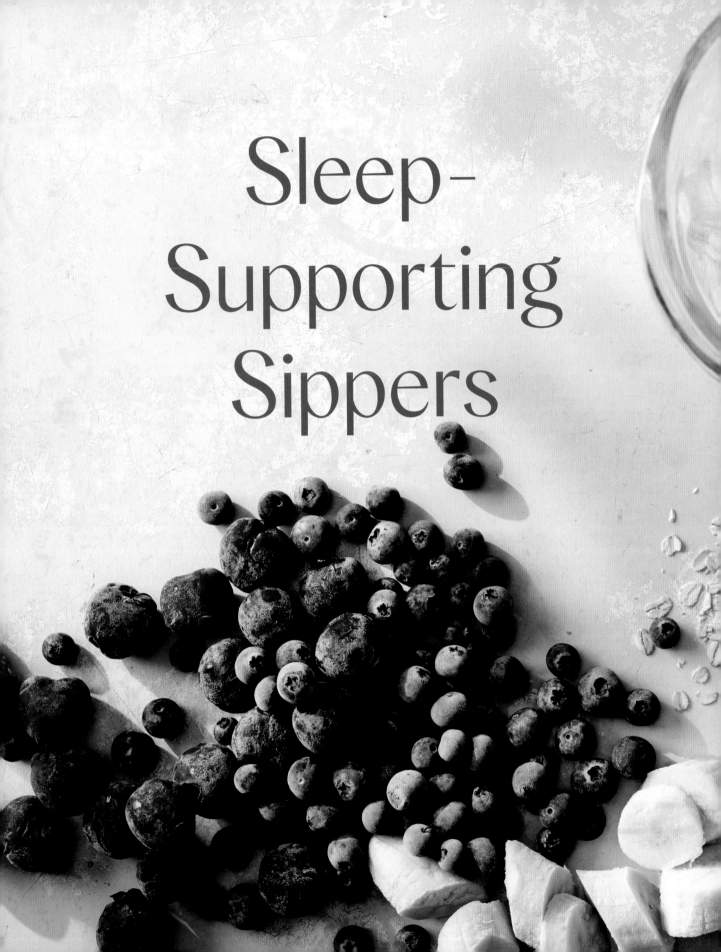

Sleep-
Supporting
Sippers

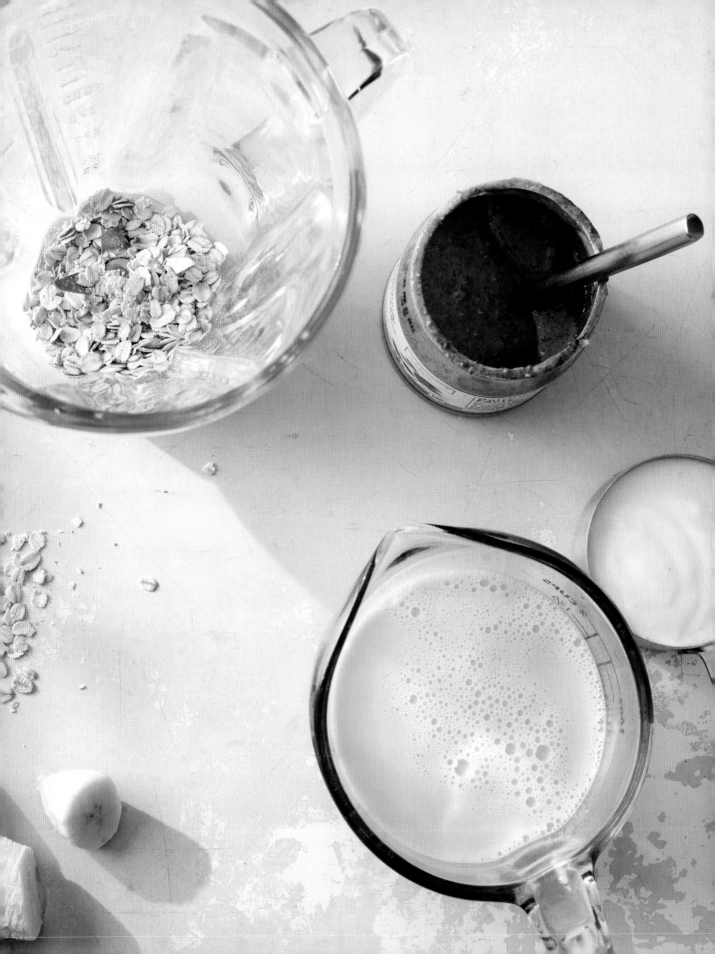

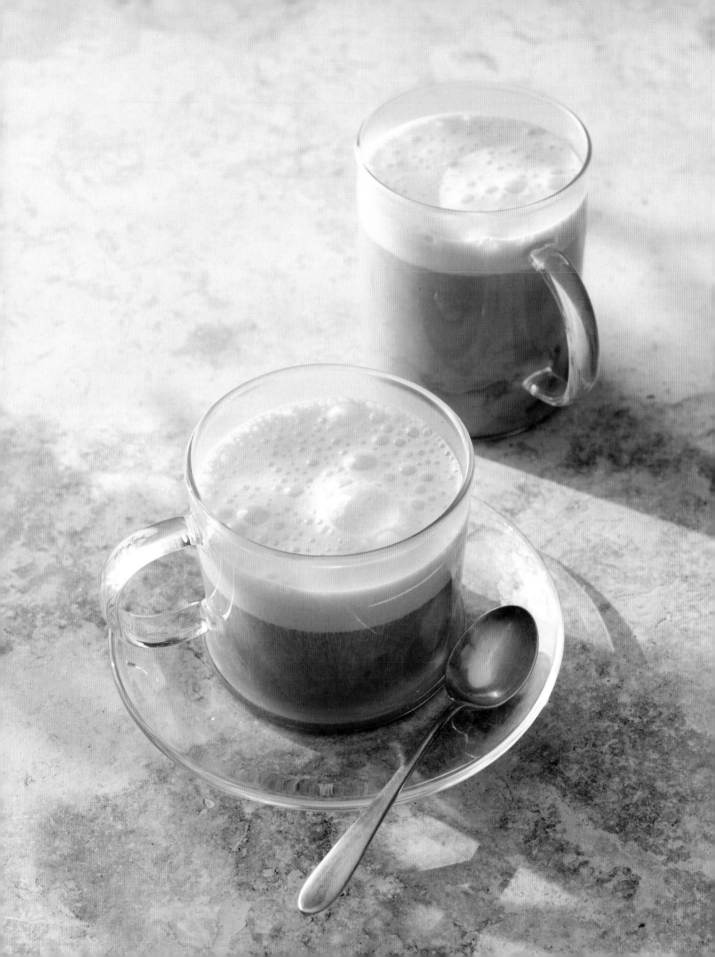

Sleepy London Fog

Serves 2 | Total Time: 15 min.

2 Earl Grey tea bags

½ cup milk

1 Tbsp. honey or maple syrup

Seeds scraped from
½ vanilla bean
(or substitute 1 tsp.
vanilla extract)

Tea leaves contain L-theanine, a nonprotein amino acid that may be helpful in the treatment of anxiety and sleep disturbances. For a late-afternoon or evening beverage, go with decaf teas to avoid disrupting your circadian rhythm with excess caffeine. Earl Grey is a widely available, bergamot-scented black tea. If you don't care for bergamot, use a plain black tea or an Indian-style masala chai blend in this recipe.

1. Place each tea bag in a mug. In a small pot, bring 1⅓ cups of water to a boil, then divide the hot water between the mugs.

2. Return the pot to the stove, add the milk, honey, and vanilla, and cook over medium-low heat, whisking frequently, just until steaming, about 5 minutes. Remove from heat, whisk vigorously to froth, then divide the mixture between the 2 mugs. Remove and discard the tea bags and serve immediately.

Gingered Stone Fruit Spritz

Serves 1	Total Time: 5 min.

Handful of ice cubes

2 Tbsp. syrup reserved from Midsummer Compote (page 98)

6 oz. (¾ cup) sparkling water

Strip of lemon peel

Sprig of fresh lemon verbena or lemon balm, for garnish (optional)

If the fruit you use to make the Midsummer Compote in our Pantry chapter is particularly juicy, consider yourself lucky! The deep crimson syrup that remains after you've eaten the cherries and plums is a beautiful concentrate for zhuzhing up fizzy low- and no-ABV beverages. For leveling up our basic spritz, go ahead and add a shot of tequila or bourbon, or swap out the sparkling water for a splash of prosecco. Just avoid going overboard on any alcohol, chase each and every cocktail with a glass of water, and—as always—don't drink too close to bedtime.

Fill a collins glass with ice, then add the syrup. Top with sparkling water, squeeze the lemon peel over the surface of the drink to express its oils, garnish with a sprig of lemon verbena, if using, and serve immediately.

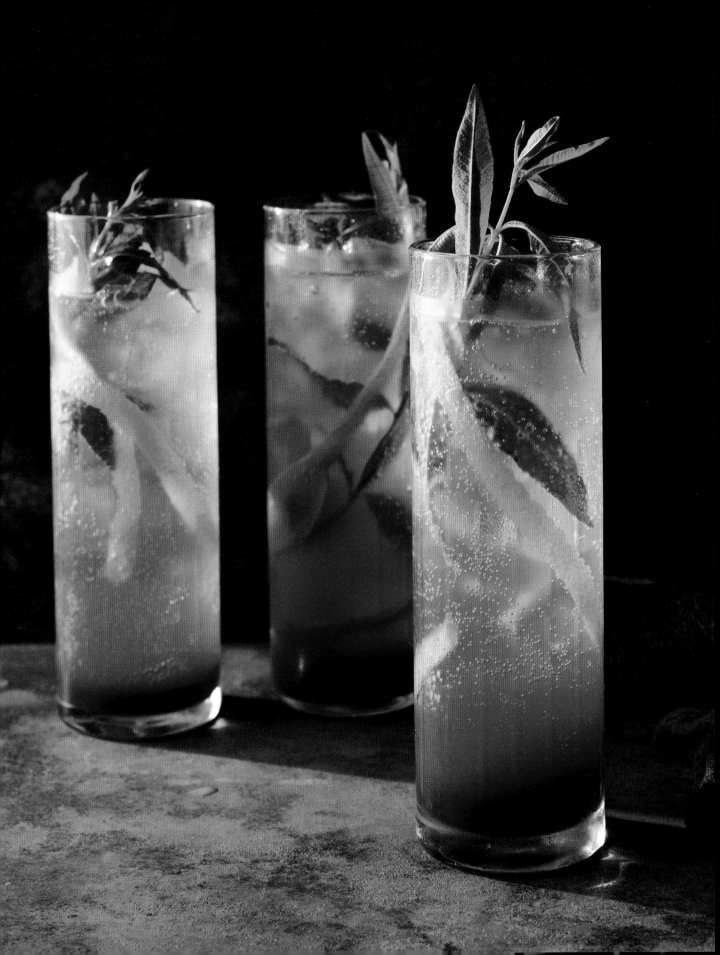

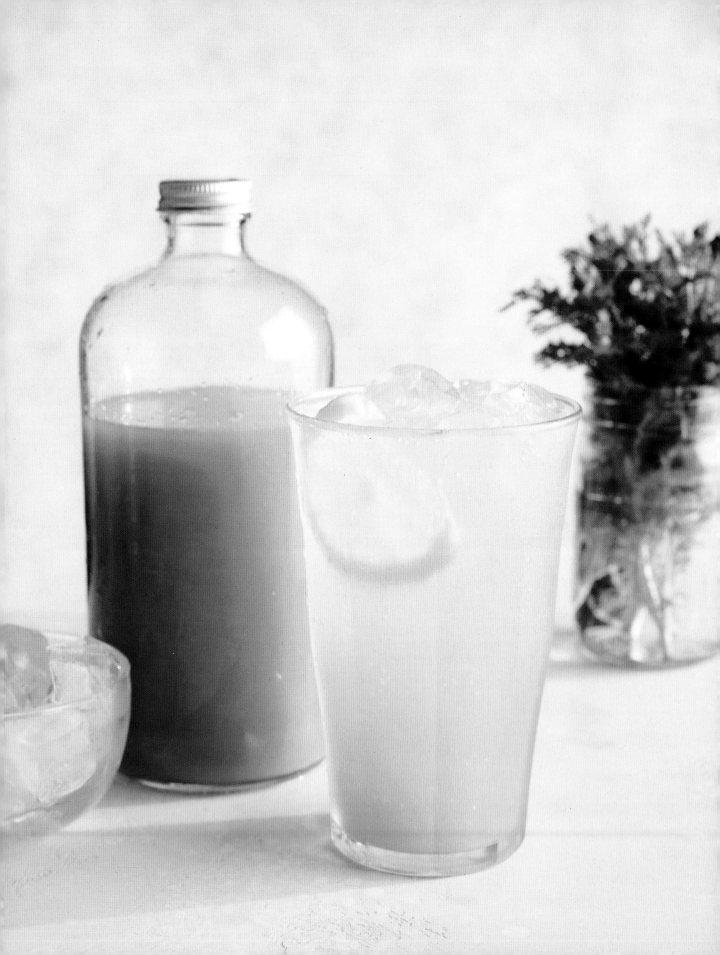

Chamomile-Ginger Cordial

Makes 3 cups

Total Time: 50 min., plus 4 hr. infusing

1 cup thinly sliced fresh ginger

²/₃ cup honey or maple syrup

8 chamomile tea bags

Historically, chamomile has been used to treat sleeplessness and anxiety, and a meta-analysis published in 2019 supports some of these effects. It's also a soothing and aromatic edible herb that lends its sweet apple-y flavor to drinks and foods. If your local farmers' market has fresh chamomile blossoms for sale, feel free to use a handful of the dainty flowers here in place of supermarket tea bags.

Enjoy a tablespoon or two of this concentrated syrup in a cold glass of soda water, stirred into warm milk or oats, or drizzled over desserts like pound cake or our Banana-Chamomile Shortcake (page 252). Or, for a gingery alcoholic treat, add a splash to a pitcher of white sangria.

1. In a medium pot, combine 5 cups of cold water, the ginger, and honey and bring to a boil over medium-high heat (don't walk away—it can boil over quickly). Lower the heat to simmer and cook, stirring occasionally, until the ginger is tender when poked with a fork, 30–35 minutes.

2. Remove the pot from heat, add the tea bags, cover, and steep at least 4 hours or overnight.

3. Remove and discard the tea bags, squeezing to extract as much liquid as possible back into the pot. Transfer the liquid and ginger to a blender and process until smooth (alternatively, submerge a hand blender directly in the pot). Strain through a fine-mesh strainer, pressing on the solids to extract as much liquid as possible; discard the solids. Decant the cordial into glass bottles or jars, cover tightly, then transfer to the fridge and use within 1 month.

The Restful Smoothie

Serves 2–4	Total Time: 10 min.

¼ cup rolled
(old-fashioned) oats

1½ cups unsweetened oat milk

1 very ripe medium banana,
peeled and frozen

1 cup frozen blueberries

½ cup frozen pitted
sour cherries

½ cup vanilla-flavored
oat yogurt

2 Tbsp. almond butter
or sunflower butter

You can't tell from looking at this super-simple recipe, but it was in fact the most difficult one for us to get just right. Marie-Pierre had a pretty specific nutritional breakdown in mind for the perfect breakfast smoothie. Kat has a background in desserts and is a stickler for consistency when it comes to milkshake-adjacent frozen beverages. By backing into an all-plant-based formula, we were able to land on a drink that's low in saturated fat, high in fiber, calcium, potassium, and antioxidants, and full of fruits shown to either increase serum melatonin (banana) or contain their own melatonin (sour cherries). A handful of soaked rolled oats provides extra fiber and also acts as a starchy emulsifier, preventing the smoothie from separating. We hope you're as happy with it as we are.

1. In a blender, combine the oats and oat milk and set aside to soak until the grains are softened and hydrated, about 5 minutes.

2. Add the banana, blueberries, cherries, yogurt, and almond butter. Blend until smooth and serve immediately.

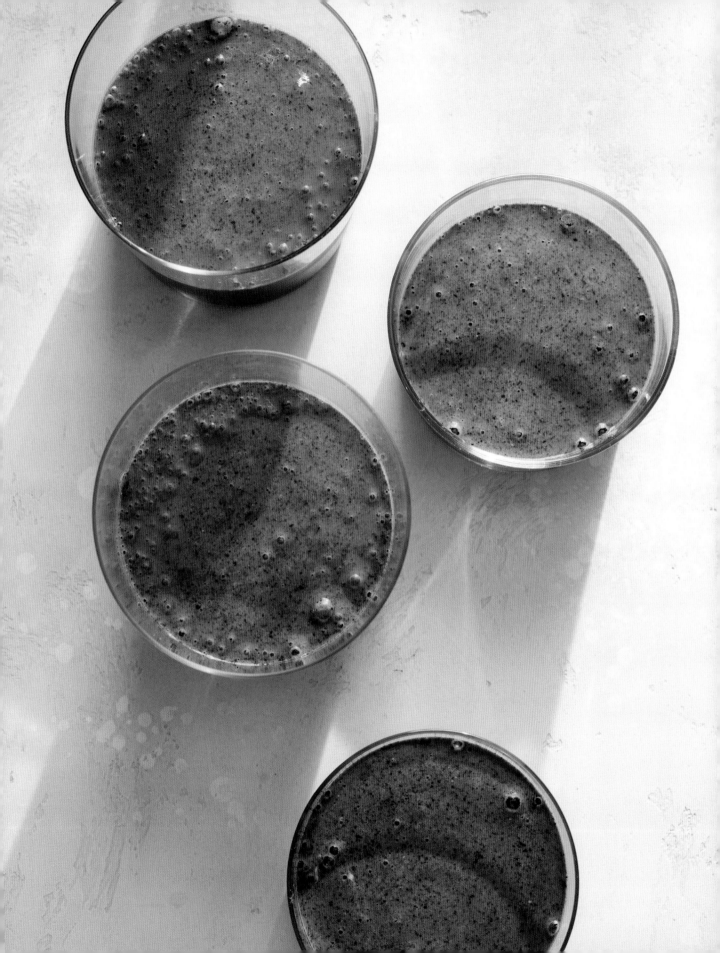

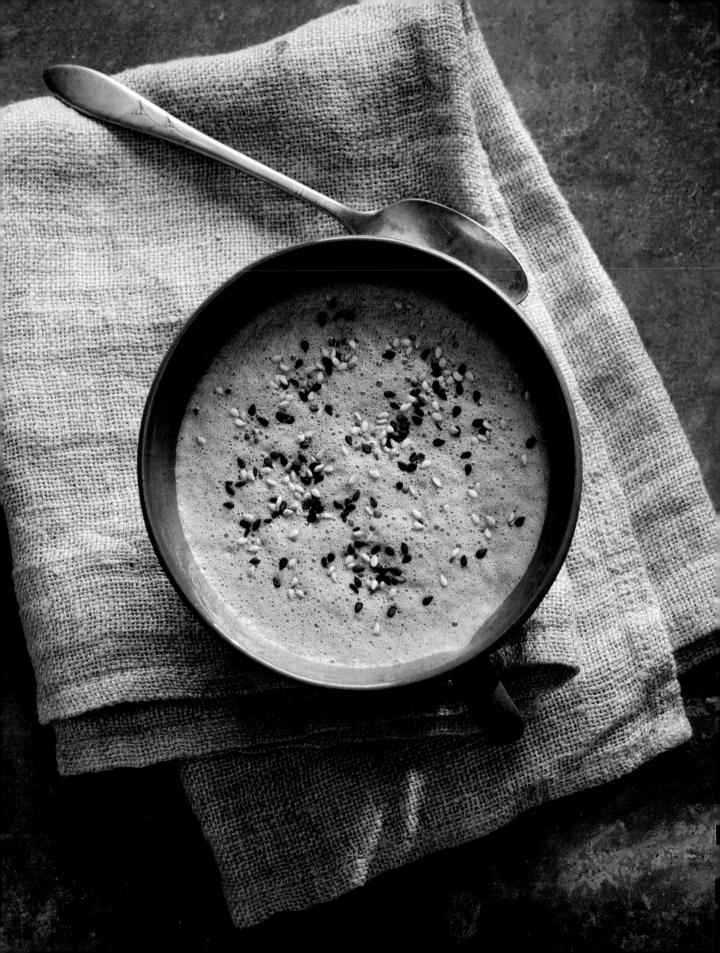

Creamy Tahini Cocoa

Serves 2	Total Time: 10 min.

¼ cup cocoa powder

2 Tbsp. maple syrup or honey

½ tsp. ground cinnamon

2 cups milk

¼ cup tahini

Pinch of kosher salt

1 tsp. toasted sesame seeds, for sprinkling (optional)

Tryptophan-rich tahini provides the richness of full-fat dairy and chocolate, but without the saturated fat. Cocoa powder brings its deep and chocolatey flavor and the health benefits of cacao without the added sugar. Enjoy this wholesome warm drink as a snack, dessert, or a mid-morning treat.

In a small pot, whisk together the cocoa powder, maple syrup, cinnamon, and ¼ cup of water. Bring to a simmer over medium heat, then whisk in the milk and tahini. Cook, stirring occasionally, until hot, then remove from heat and whisk vigorously to froth the liquid. Ladle into 2 mugs, sprinkle with salt and sesame seeds, if using, and serve warm.

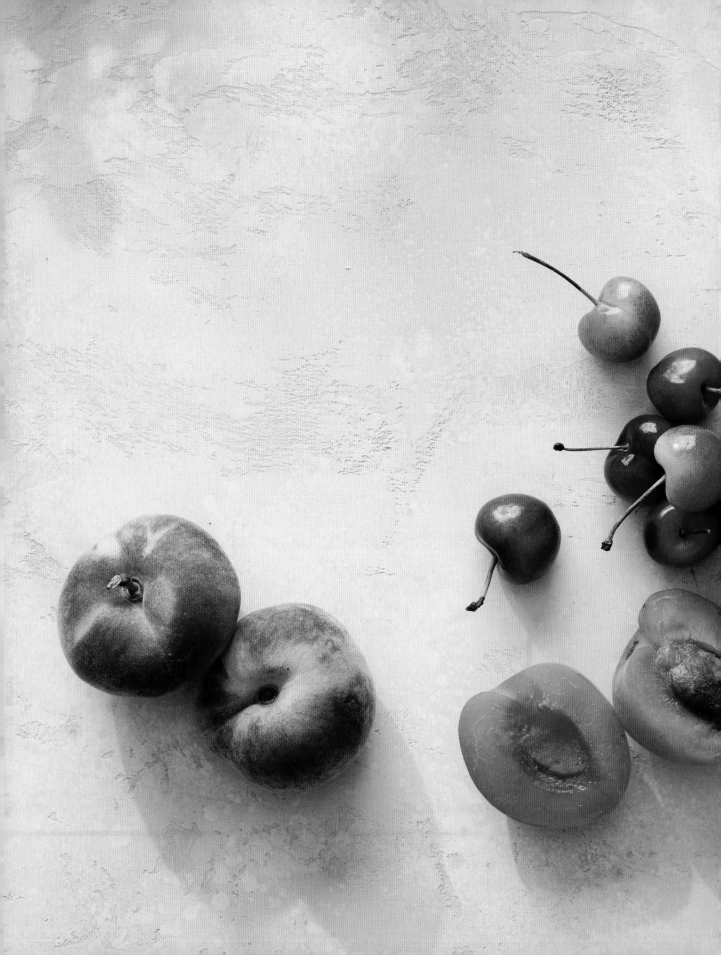

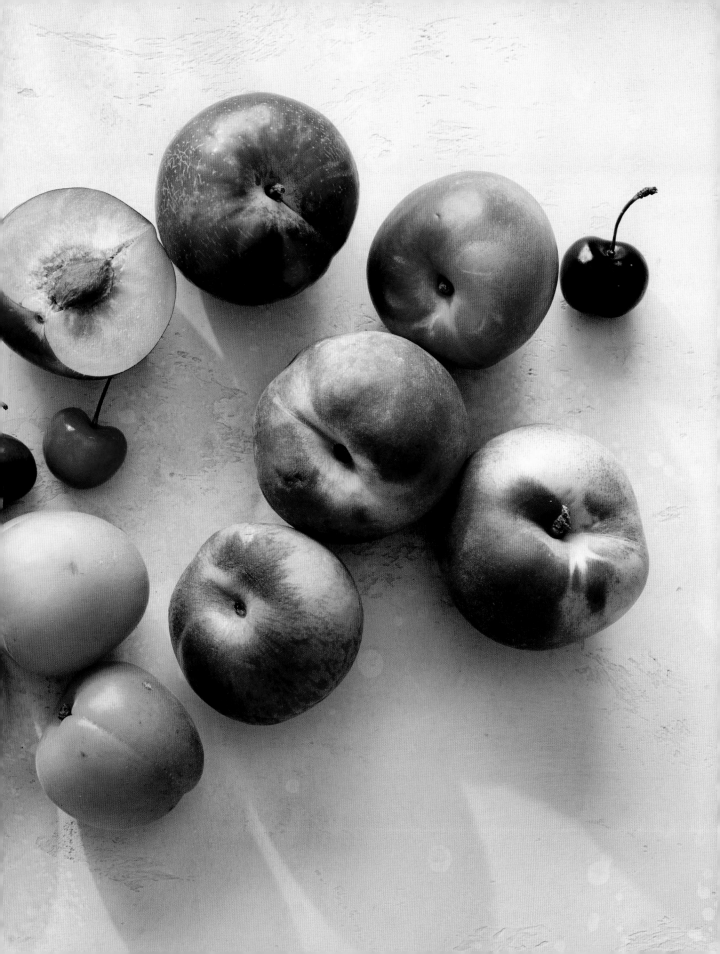

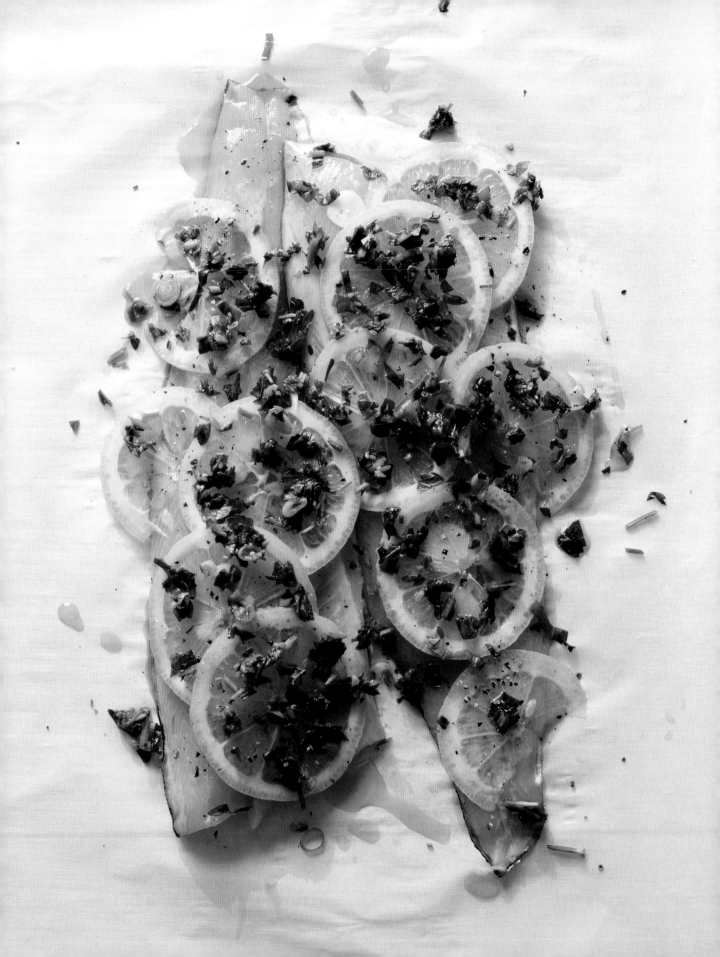

Resources for Food and Sleep

FOOD

In addition to the usual big-name online delivery services for groceries, fresh foods, and special ingredients, here are a few more of our favorite online sources.

www.burlapandbarrel.com

The team behind this public benefit corporation scours the world for small family farms growing exceptional herbs and spices, then partners with them directly to bring consumers exceptionally fresh, high-quality ingredients and also offer growers a fair living wage. Check back regularly, as new single-origin spices and custom blends are being added to their lineup all the time.

www.foodsofnations.com

Kalustyan's is a favorite independently owned retailer of New York chefs and home cooks. It's a terrific source for spices, seeds, nuts, and other specialty ingredients and they ship their excellent selection nationwide.

www.fultonfishmarket.com

If you don't have access to great seafood in your area, New York City's Fulton Fish Market is a reliable mail-order option. Deliveries are overnighted on dry ice.

www.kingarthurbaking.com

King Arthur offers a robust assortment of whole grain flour direct to consumers. (Once you've stocked up, be sure to check out the brand's extensive online recipe library.)

www.mariani.com

While it's *possible* to find most foods just about any time of the year, off-season produce can be lacking in flavor and nutrition (and is less sustainable than eating locally and in-season). For the winter months, stock your pantry with high-quality dried fruit, which is typically harvested and processed at peak ripeness. If your local market doesn't have a good selection, check out California brand Mariani, which offers a lovely assortment of dried tropical and orchard fruits, raisins, and dried berries.

www.melissas.com

If you don't have a great source for fresh fruits, vegetables, and herbs near you, treat yourself to some of Melissa's online selection. The LA-based specialty produce distributor is the largest in the United States and is a reliable source for a whole rainbow of sleep-supporting foods from near and far.

www.mercato.com

For general grocery deliveries, we like the online service Mercato, which works directly with local, independent supermarkets, butcher shops, and other independent food businesses.

www.pikeplacefish.com

Seattle's Pike Place Fish Market is an excellent source for fresh and frozen Pacific seafood like Alaskan salmon, halibut, and crab.

SLEEP

Sleep Organizations

American Academy of Sleep Medicine: www.aasm.org
If you're looking for an accredited sleep medicine specialist or clinic, the patient resources on the AASM website offer a directory of providers. You'll also find information on topics like sleep apnea and other disorders, and much more.

National Sleep Foundation: www.thensf.org
This nonprofit offers science-based resources on their website, including articles on a broad range of sleep topics, from up-to-date research to tips on improving your sleep quality.

Society of Behavioral Sleep Medicine: www.behaviorialsleep.org
If you are looking for a clinician who specializes in cognitive behavioral therapy to manage sleep disorders, you'll find accredited providers on this site, as well as other resources on the behavioral sleep medicine approach to treatment.

Sleep Apps

Haleo is an "online sleep clinic" that uses cognitive behavioral therapy for insomnia treatment as well as for shift workers dealing with sleep problems. It also offers a "sleep optimization program." The information and techniques provided are science-based and clinically proven. Find it in app stores for iOS and Android.

References

INTRODUCTION

Kansagra, Sujay. "Sleep Disorders in Adolescents." *Pediatrics* 145, no. 2 (May 2020): S204–S209. https://doi.org/10.1542/peds.2019-2056I.

Medic, Goran, et al. "Short- and Long-Term Health Consequences of Sleep Disruption." *Nature and Science of Sleep* 9 (May 2017): 151–161. https://doi.org/10.2147%2FNSS.S134864.

St-Onge, Marie-Pierre, et al. "Short Sleep Duration Increases Energy Intakes but Does Not Change Energy Expenditure in Normal-Weight Individuals." *The American Journal of Clinical Nutrition* 94, no. 2 (2011): 410–416. https://doi.org/10.3945/ajcn.111.013904.

St-Onge, Marie-Pierre, et al. "Sleep Restriction Leads to Increased Activation of Brain Regions Sensitive to Food Stimuli." *The American Journal of Clinical Nutrition* 95, no. 4 (2012): 818–824. https://doi.org/10.3945/ajcn.111.027383.

Tasali, Esra, et al. "Effect of Sleep Extension on Objectively Assessed Energy Intake Among Adults with Overweight in Real-life Settings: A Randomized Clinical Trial." *JAMA Internal Medicine* 182, no. 4 (2022): 365–374. https://doi.org/10.1001/jamainternmed.2021.8098.

CHAPTER 1

Afaghi, Ahmad, et al. "High-Glycemic-Index Carbohydrate Meals Shorten Sleep Onset," *The American Journal of Clinical Nutrition* 85, no. 2 (2007): 426–430. https://doi.org/10.1093/ajcn/85.2.426.

Albanes, Demetrius, et al. "Alpha-Tocopherol and Beta-Carotene Supplements and Lung Cancer Incidence in the Alpha-Tocopherol, Beta-Carotene Cancer Prevention Study: Effects of Base-Line Characteristics and Study Compliance." *Journal of the National Cancer Institute* 88, no. 21 (1996): 1560–1570. https://doi.org/10.1093/jnci/88.21.1560.

The Alpha-Tocopherol Beta Carotene Cancer Prevention Study Group. "The Effect of Vitamin E and Beta Carotene on the Incidence of Lung Cancer and Other Cancers in Male Smokers." *New England Journal of Medicine* 330 (1994): 1029–1035. https://doi.org/10.1056/NEJM199404143301501.

Castro-Diehl, Cecilia, et al. "Mediterranean Diet Pattern and Sleep Duration and Insomnia Symptoms in the Multi-Ethnic Study of Atherosclerosis." *Sleep* 41, no. 11 (2018). https://doi.org/10.1093/sleep/zsy158.

Gao, Qi, et al. "The Association between Vitamin D Deficiency and Sleep Disorders: A Systematic Review and Meta-Analysis." *Nutrients* 10, no. 10 (October 2018): 1395. https://doi.org/10.3390/nu10101395.

Murat, Semiz, et al. "Assessment of Subjective Sleep Quality in Iron Deficiency Anaemia." *African Health Sciences* 15, no. 2 (2015): 621–627. https://doi.org/10.4314/ahs.v15i2.40.

Shechter, Ari, et al. "Alterations in Sleep Architecture in Response to Experimental Sleep Curtailment Are Associated with Signs of Positive Energy Balance." *American Journal of Physiology: Regulatory, Integrative and Comparative Physiology* 303, no. 9 (2012): R883–9. https://doi.org/10.1152/ajpregu.00222.2012.

St-Onge, Marie-Pierre, et al. "Fiber and Saturated Fat Are Associated with Sleep Arousals and Slow Wave Sleep." *Journal of Clinical Sleep Medicine* 12, no. 1 (2016): 19–24. https://doi.org/10.5664/jcsm.5384.

St-Onge, Marie-Pierre, et al. "Sleep Restriction Increases the Neuronal Response to Unhealthy Food in Normal-Weight Individuals." *International Journal of Obesity* 38, no. 3 (2014): 411–416. https://doi.org/10.1038/ijo.2013.114.

St-Onge, Marie-Pierre, et al. "Sleep Restriction Leads to Increased Activation of Brain Regions Sensitive to Food Stimuli." *The American Journal of Clinical Nutrition* 95, no. 4 (2012): 818–824. https://doi.org/10.3945/ajcn.111.027383.

CHAPTER 2

Avni, Tomer, et al. "Iron Supplementation for Restless Legs Syndrome—A Systematic Review and Meta-Analysis." *European Journal of Internal Medicine* 63 (2019): 34–41. https//doi.org/10.1016/j.ejim.2019.02.009.

Casas, Irene, et al. "Effects of a Mediterranean Diet Intervention on Maternal Stress, Well-Being, and Sleep Quality throughout Gestation—The IMPACT-BCN Trial." *Nutrients* 15, no. 10 (May 2023): 2362. https://doi.org/10.3390/nu15102362.

Chellappa, Sarah L., et al. "Daytime Eating Prevents Internal Circadian Misalignment and Glucose Intolerance in Night Work." *Science Advances* 7, no. 49 (2021): eabg9910. https://doi.org/10.1126/sciadv.abg9910.

Duraccio, Kara McRae, et al. "Losing Sleep by Staying Up Late Leads Adolescents to Consume More Carbohydrates and a Higher Glycemic Load." *Sleep* 45, no. 3 (March 2022): zsab269. https://doi.org/10.1093/sleep/zsab269.

Flor-Alemany, Marta, et al. "Associations of Mediterranean Diet with Psychological Ill-Being And Well-Being throughout the Pregnancy Course: The GESTAFIT Project." *Quality of Life Research* 31, no. 9 (2022): 2705–2716. https://doi.org/10.1007/s11136-022-03121-2.

Gangwisch, James E., et al. "High Glycemic Index and Glycemic Load Diets as Risk Factors for Insomnia: Analyses from the Women's Health Initiative." *The American Journal of Clinical Nutrition* 111, no. 2 (2020): 429–439. https://doi.org/10.1093/ajcn/nqz275.

Georgoulis, Michael, et al. "Dose-Response Relationship Between Weight Loss and Improvements in Obstructive Sleep Apnea Severity After a Diet/Lifestyle Interventions: Secondary Analyses of the 'MIMOSA' Randomized Clinical Trial." *Journal of Clinical Sleep Medicine* 18, no. 5 (2022): 1251–1261. https://doi.org/10.5664/jcsm.9834.

Her, Jihoo, and Mi-Kyoung Cho. "Effect of Aromatherapy on Sleep Quality of Adults and Elderly People: A Systematic Literature Review and Meta-Analysis." *Complementary Therapies in Medicine* 60 (2021): 102739. https://doi.org/10.1016/j.ctim.2021.102739.

Karbasi, Samira, et al. "Association Between Adherence to the Dietary Approaches to Stop Hypertension (DASH) Diet and Maternal and Infant Sleep Disorders." *BMC Nutrition* 8, no. 1 (September 2022): 103. https://doi.org/10.1186/s40795-022-00600-0.

Makarem, Nour, et al. "Habitual Nightly Fasting Duration, Eating Timing, and Eating Frequency Are Associated with Cardiometabolic Risk in Women." *Nutrients* 12, no. 10 (October 2020): 3043. https://doi.org/10.3390/nu12103043.

Makarem, Nour, et al. "Rest-Activity Rhythms Are Associated With Prevalent Cardiovascular Disease, Hypertension, Obesity, and Central Adiposity in a Nationally Representative Sample of US Adults." *Journal of the American Heart Association* 13, no. 1 (2024): e032073. https://doi.org/10.1161/JAHA.122.032073.

Manoogian, Emily N. C., et al. "Time-Restricted Eating for the Prevention and Management of Metabolic Diseases." *Endocrine Reviews* 43, no. 2 (2022): 405–436. https://doi.org/10.1210/endrev/bnab027.

Melaku, Yohannes Adama, et al. "High-Quality and Anti-Inflammatory Diets and a Healthy Lifestyle Are Associated with Lower Sleep Apnea Risk." *Journal of Clinical Sleep Medicine* 18, no. 6 (2022): 1667–1679. https://doi.org/10.5664/jcsm.9950.

The Multi-Ethnic Study of Atherosclerosis (MESA). https://internal.mesa-nhlbi.org/.

Qian, Jingyi, et al. "Daytime Eating Prevents Mood Vulnerability in Night Work." *Proceedings of the National Academy of Sciences of the United States of America* 119, no. 38 (2022): e2206348119. https://doi.org/10.1073/pnas.2206348119.

St-Onge, Marie-Pierre, et al. "Impact of Change in Bedtime Variability on Body Composition and Inflammation: Secondary Findings from the Go Red for Women Strategically Focused Research Network." *International Journal Of Obesity* 44, no. 8 (2020): 1803–1806. https://doi.org/10.1038/s41366-020-0555-1.

Tang, Yueheng, et al. "The Therapeutic Effect of Aromatherapy on Insomnia: A Meta-Analysis." *Journal of Affective Disorders.* 288 (2021): 1–9. https://doi.org/10.1016/j.jad.2021.03.066.

Vallat, Raphael, et al. "How People Wake Up Is Associated with Previous Night's Sleep Together with Physical Activity and Food Intake." *Nature Communications* 13, no. 1 (November 2022): 7116. https://doi.org/10.1038/s41467-022-34503-2.

Wallace, Danielle A., et al. "Associations Between Evening Shift Work, Irregular Sleep Timing, and Gestational Diabetes in the Nulliparous Pregnancy Outcomes Study: Monitoring Mothers-to-Be (nuMoM2b)." *Sleep* 46, no. 4 (2023): zsac297. https://doi.org/10.1093/sleep/zsac297.

Wallace, Danielle A., et al. "Rest-Activity Rhythms Across the Lifespan: Cross-Sectional Findings from the US Representative National Health and Nutrition Examination Survey." *Sleep* 46, no. 11 (2023): zsad220. https://doi.org/10.1093/sleep/zsad220.

Wang, Monica L., et al. "Sugar-Sweetened Beverage Consumption and Sleep Duration and Quality Among Pregnant Women." *Journal of Nutrition Education and Behavior* 53, no. 9 (2021): 793–797. https://doi.org/10.1016/j.jneb.2021.02.010.

Zerón-Rugerio, María Fernanda, et al. "Eating Jet Lag: A Marker of the Variability in Meal Timing and Its Association with Body Mass Index." *Nutrients* 11, no. 12 (December 2019): 2980. https://doi.org10.3390/nu11122980.

CHAPTER 3

St-Onge, Marie-Pierre, et al. "Fiber and Saturated Fat Are Associated with Sleep Arousals and Slow Wave Sleep." *Journal of Clinical Sleep Medicine* 12, no. 1 (2016): 19–24. https://doi.org/10.5664/jcsm.5384.

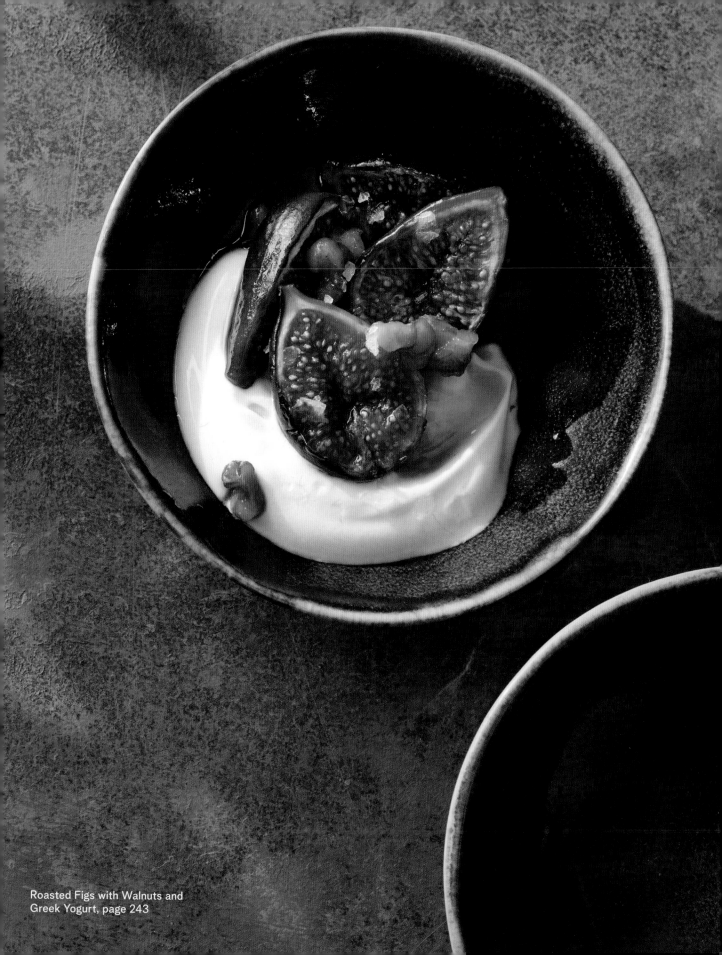

Roasted Figs with Walnuts and
Greek Yogurt, page 243

Acknowledgments

This book would not have been possible without our agent, Kitty Cowles, who had the spark of inspiration that brought this dream team together. Thank you for your guidance through this process, your encouragement, and your patience. Thanks also to Becky Cabaza, for helping us shape and fine-tune decades of research into an inviting and actionable road map to a well-rested, healthier life. You were such a delight to work with!

A big thanks to our editor, Doris Cooper, for being our number one cheerleader and believing in this book, for pushing us to deliver the best product possible; to Katie McClimon, for the cheerful air traffic control; and the full team at Simon & Schuster: Richard Rhorer, Elizabeth Breeden, Stacy Reichgott, Jessica Preeg, Jen Wang, Jan Derevjanik, Jessie McNiel, Laura Jarrett, Beth Maglione. Your professionalism and dedication made the publishing process so rewarding.

Thank you to our hugely talented art team: David Malosh, your photography, and Simon Andrews, your food styling, made our recipes sparkle on the page. And Paige Hicks, thank you for opening up your studio and staggering prop collection for this project. Working with all of you was such a wonderful experience!

To Kat, my partner in this project. Thank you for your creativity in designing delicious recipes and opening the culinary world to me. Your talent and passion are inspirational.

To my friends and colleagues, who have advised, reassured, and supported me in this project and who make me happy to come to work every day, and all of the research assistants, students, and interns who have worked in my lab over the years. To my colleagues in sleep, nutrition, and obesity, and everyone at the AHA: You make this work so worthwhile.

To my mom and dad, for the sacrifices you've made that opened so many doors for me. Thank you for being such great role models and encouraging me to work hard and follow my own path.

And to my husband, Michael, and twins, Jacob and Sarah, for taste-testing every recipe and being my so-very-most honest critics! Thank you for keeping me grounded and pushing me to go beyond my comfort zone. Without you, I wouldn't have such a fun, well-rounded work-life balance. I love you so very much. —M-P

Thanks to my brilliant coauthor, Marie-Pierre; to my steadfast taste tester and kitty coparent, Kate; and my funniest and my most fabulous friend, Joey. And of course, thanks and love, as always, to Mom & Dad. xo —KC

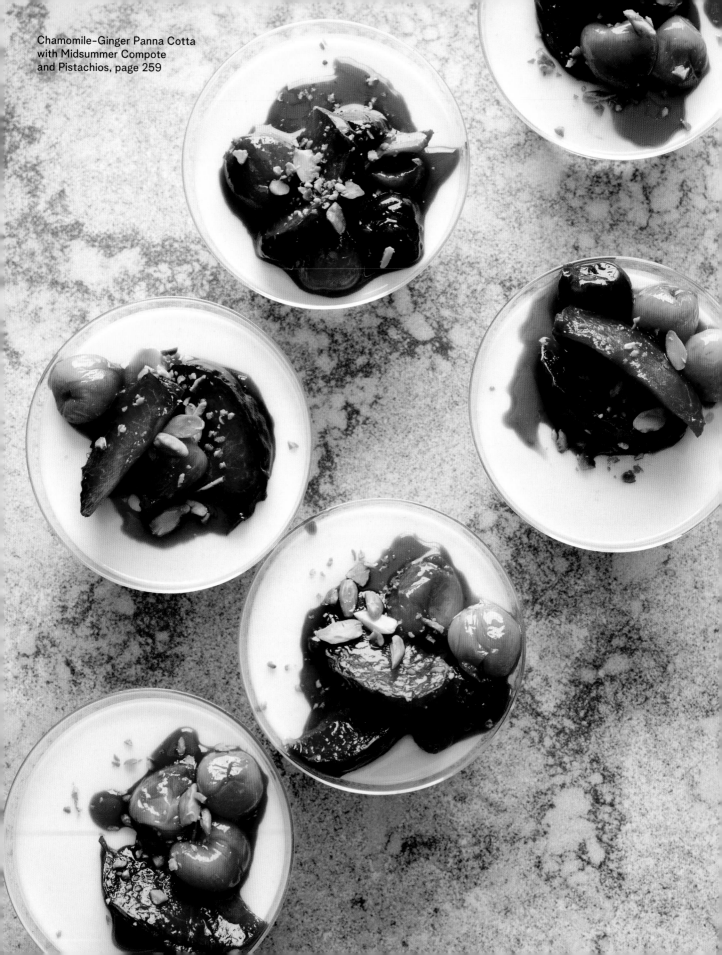

Chamomile–Ginger Panna Cotta
with Midsummer Compote
and Pistachios, page 259

Index

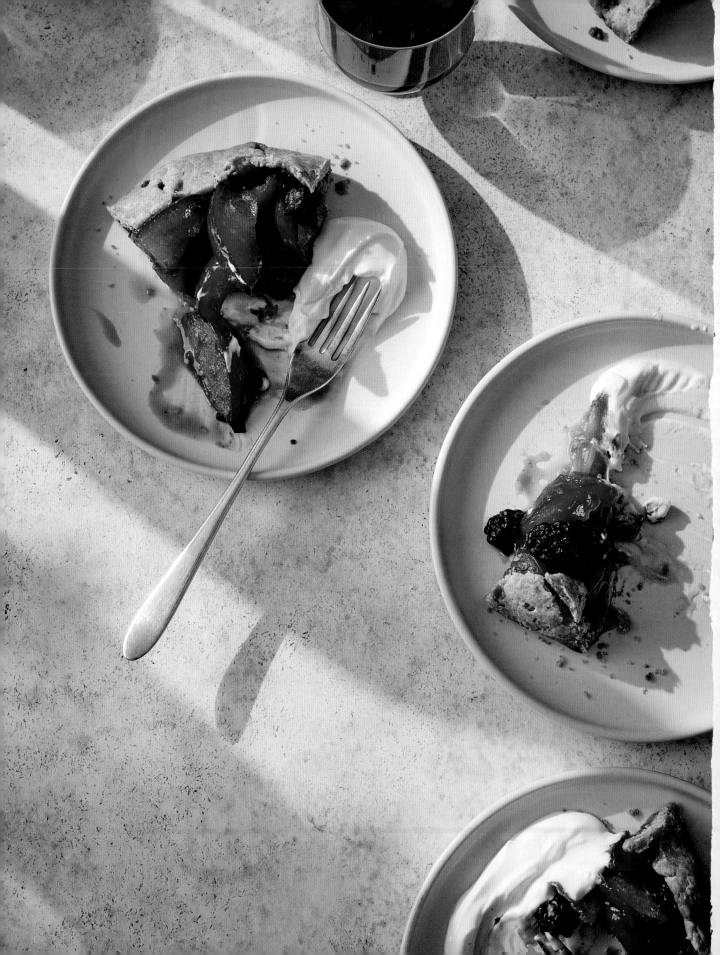